THIS IS VEGAN
PROPAGANDA

THIS IS VEGAN PROPAGANDA

(AND OTHER LIES THE MEAT INDUSTRY TELLS YOU)

ED WINTERS

Vermilion
LONDON

Vermilion, an imprint of Ebury Publishing,
20 Vauxhall Bridge Road,
London SW1V 2SA

Vermilion is part of the Penguin Random House group of companies
whose addresses can be found at global.penguinrandomhouse.com

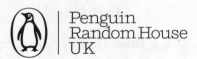

Copyright © Ed Winters 2022

Ed Winters has asserted his right to be identified as the
author of this Work in accordance with the Copyright,
Designs and Patents Act 1988

Editorial Consultant: Paul Murphy

First published by Vermilion in 2022

www.penguin.co.uk

A CIP catalogue record for this book is available from
the British Library

ISBN 9781785043765

Printed and bound in Great Britain by Clays Ltd, Elcograf S.p.A.

The authorised representative in the EEA is Penguin Random House
Ireland, Morrison Chambers, 32 Nassau Street, Dublin D02 YH68

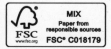

Penguin Random House is committed to a
sustainable future for our business, our readers
and our planet. This book is made from Forest
Stewardship Council® certified paper.

CONTENTS

CONTENTS

INTRODUCTION

When you read the word 'vegan', what are the first thoughts that come into your head? If I'd been asked that question eight years ago, I would have told you, 'Vegans are extremists, with no sense of humour, who should mind their own business and stop forcing their views on people, not to mention they're arrogant, self-righteous, judgemental and militant.' I would then have gone on to say, 'I have nothing against vegans, I just wish they would stop trying to make other people vegan and respect my personal choice to eat meat. And besides, meat tastes too good to give up.'

The word 'vegan' is currently one of the most emotive there is. Love it or hate it, its ability to elicit a response cannot be denied. However, despite the word being so divisive, often very little is known about the enormous impact of animal consumption. So this is not only the book that I wish I could have given myself many years ago when I had a strong opinion of veganism while knowing very little about it or people's motivations for embracing it, but it is also a comprehensive resource for vegans who want to better understand the arguments that people use against veganism and why they use them, as well as how to respond to them and become more effective advocates in the process.

It's no secret that veganism is growing all over the world and has become one of the most prevalent and discussed social movements of this generation. But while most of us will be aware that the primary motivations for people going vegan and adopting plant-based diets include animal rights, the environment, pandemic prevention and personal health, often little is known about the complexity and true scale of these issues, which is exactly what this book aims to do: lay out the enormity of the injustice that is animal exploitation.

Every time we eat, we have the power to radically transform the world we live in and simultaneously contribute to addressing many of the most pressing issues that our species currently faces: climate change, infectious disease, chronic disease, human exploitation and, of course, non-human exploitation. Every single day, our choices can help alleviate all of these problems or they can perpetuate them.

I think it's important to state that conversations about veganism and animal rights can often lead to feelings of judgement, but the purpose of this book is not to demonise people who eat meat, dairy and eggs, or who work in the animal industries. Quite the contrary in fact. I don't for one moment believe that they are all bad people. Good people can do bad things. Each and every one of us is a testament to that. I also believe that knowledge is power and when we are given both sides of the story we are then able to make informed decisions for ourselves. The problem is that we haven't been given both sides of the story – the reality of animal farming is hidden from us or disguised by marketing labels and industry PR.

Ironically, while the animal farming industries hide the reality of how animal products are produced behind labels, they also disregard the other side of the story as simply being 'vegan propaganda'. This catch-all phrase is used to discredit anything that challenges them, no matter how strong the evidence or solid the moral argument. I have written this book to offer this other side, supported by scientific studies, which are all referenced in case you want to find out more. I hope that it will equip you, the reader, with the knowledge to make informed decisions about your own actions and that it will make you feel empowered, because we all have a say in influencing what the future will look like. It is the amalgamation of six years of research, reading and conversations that I have had with people from every part of the spectrum, from slaughterhouse workers and farmers to animal rights philosophers, environmentalists and everyday consumers. It has been a journey that has so far involved me debating veganism on live television in front of millions of people, giving hundreds of speeches and lectures, and visiting farms and slaughterhouses around the world.

However, this book goes beyond just making the case for veganism and explores the psychological and social mechanisms behind why we do what we do, highlighting and exposing the societal and cultural constructs that create passive complicity in industries that, on deeper evaluation, contradict the fundamental values that we live by. In essence, this book discusses a myriad of ideas and themes in the hope of empowering vegans to feel more educated and confident in discussing why they are vegan, while at the same time being a comprehensive resource for those looking to learn more about veganism. I hope this prompts questions and highlights information that can in turn act as catalysts for self-reflection that ultimately leads to us challenging our own habits, unconscious or otherwise.

Some of the information and topics I cover in this book make for uncomfortable reading. Realising the scale of mass suffering and death that is relentlessly occurring every second of the day is by far the hardest aspect to face. To put it into perspective, it is estimated that globally around 220 million land animals are killed for food every day,[1] and when you factor in marine animals that number increases to somewhere between 2.4 and 6.3 billion.[2] Every. Single. Day. That means that somewhere between 28,000 and 73,000 animals are killed every second, a completely incomprehensible number.

When we talk about animal exploitation, the scale is absolutely staggering. But it's not just the scale, it's the practices that are carried out on these individuals, each with their own experiences and emotions, all suffering as a result of what we are doing to them. Non-human animals are the oppressed majority, each and every one of them at the mercy of our dominance, intellect and strength.

We have created a form of tyranny over the natural world, pillaging, extracting, using and destroying as we please. We have placed ourselves above the ecological life support systems that our species depends on for survival and exploited them for our own short-term benefit, cutting down forests and polluting rivers and oceans. We have destroyed millions of years of evolution in the blink of an eye, quite literally bulldozing our way around this finite planet. For all of our intelligence, we have still failed to grasp the simple reality that we need the planet more than the planet needs us.

And as we have killed more and more animals, and destroyed more and more of the world, we have become sicker and sicker. While some people die early from having too much, others die from having too little. Preventable chronic diseases and preventable world hunger are growing in tandem, and people are suffering because of our woefully illogical, unfair and unsustainable food system. Humanity is at a crossroads: we can either continue as we currently are or set off in a new direction, learning from our previous mistakes and working for the benefit of all life.

Aristotle said, 'The roots of education are bitter, but the fruit is sweet.' Undeniably, the issues of animal exploitation, climate change and disease are bitter issues to learn about, but the potential benefits of doing so cannot be overstated. It is quite literally a matter of life and death. So, while we may say that ignorance is bliss, in reality aligning our morals and values with our actions, and in doing so creating a more peaceful, sustainable and safe world, is far more blissful than turning a blind eye to the suffering that animals are forced to endure and the catastrophic damage caused as a consequence.

As consumers we have the right to know what we are paying for, and as active participants in the exploitation of animals we also have a moral obligation to confront the truth about the choices we make. The reality is that we all have our part to play in overcoming injustice, especially one so ubiquitous, systemic and universally perpetuated as the oppression of non-human animals. With the continuing industrialisation of animal farming and the increasing number of animals being farmed, coupled with the ever-growing existential threat of climate change and future pandemics, it has never been more important to address our current food system and challenge ourselves as individuals and consumers. By doing this, we can then challenge the normalisation of our dominion over non-human animals and the natural world that in turn negatively impacts every life on this planet, ours included. Fundamentally, that's what this book is: an attempt to hold up a mirror to the absurdity of what we are doing and reveal the solution that is right there in front of us.

Non-vegans often say, 'Please stop trying to force me to be vegan,' and although this book is aimed at anyone interested in veganism, including vegans themselves who want to become more knowledgeable and better equipped for conversations with others about veganism, I can imagine that some of you who are reading this book are doing so because you have a particularly vocal family member or friend. Someone who is desperate for you to become vegan and has asked you to read it. Truth be told, throughout writing this book, I have always kept the reluctant reader in mind, the sceptic who would need the most convincing; after all, that was the person I used to be.

If that is you, then first, thank you for choosing to read this book. But second, at the end of the day, nobody can force anyone to be vegan. When you put this book down, what you choose to buy in a supermarket is entirely up to you. We often joke about the existence of the vegan police but ultimately a vegan isn't going to jump out of the cow's milk fridge and force the oat milk into your hand, and, even if they did, you could just put it down again. However, it is my wish to offer a perspective that helps you to understand veganism better, that answers the questions that you have often pondered, addresses the justifications that you have often used to defend not being vegan and ultimately encourages you to pick up the oat milk because you want to.

PART ONE

IT'S A QUESTION OF MORALITY

1.

VEGANISM IS THE MORAL BASELINE

Like nearly every vegan I have ever met, I never expected when I was younger that I would one day stop consuming all animal products. In fact, growing up, even the concept of vegetarianism was routinely a joke around the family dinner table (it's always easier to laugh at something you don't understand) with veganism only being spared because we had never heard of it. We would make truly terrible jokes, such as, 'What's the best thing about having a vegetarian around for dinner?' There would then be a pause before one of us said, 'More meat for us!' Although, truth be told, since going vegan I have encountered worse, such as the much used 'How do you know when someone is vegan? Don't worry, they'll tell you!' I know people say that vegans don't have a sense of humour but let's be honest – we're not often presented with the best material.

When I was about 12 years old, I was in an English class and my teacher asked a question along the lines of, 'What do you think about vegetarians?' I rather abruptly thrust my hand in the air and, when called on, said, 'All vegetarians are pale, weak and skinny.' It was somewhat ironic, as I ate meat every day and yet I was definitely among the weakest and skinniest in the class. I remember there then being a weirdly ominous silence. I looked at my teacher, expecting to hear, 'Well done, Edward. Great answer.' Instead, I was met with a bemused expression. I turned to look at a girl who was sitting diagonally behind me. She was a vegetarian, and I remember thinking she would validate my answer. After all, she would know better than anyone else the compromises she was making in order to pursue her values. Instead, I was met with a ferocious stare that caused me to feel very confused. It wasn't my intention to be offensive; I had merely stated what I believed to be true – or, more importantly, what I had been told was true.

As children, we are unable to rationalise and understand the dangers of the world, so we accept at face value what we are told by our parents and authority figures. From an evolutionary perspective, this makes complete sense. In prehistoric times, we were told 'Don't eat this berry,' 'Avoid this animal,' 'Don't touch the fire,' and we listened because trusting our communities was instrumental to our survival. As a child, I too was told to not touch fire because it would burn me, I was instructed not to talk to strangers as it was dangerous, and I was informed that we need meat for protein. But while pigs, cows and chickens are food, dogs and cats are pets. When I grew up and realised for myself the risks of touching fire and talking to strangers, the validation of those truths consequently validated everything else I had been told: protein comes from meat, but only a few species of animals are food, while the others are not. This sort of uncontested trust becomes particularly problematic when it inadvertently perpetuates fallacies and ideas that are now outdated and should be challenged or leads to the sorts of flawed arguments that I hear people use on a daily basis to justify their consumption of animal products.

In that moment in the classroom when I was 12 years old, I was simply regurgitating information that I had been told my entire life: if we stop eating meat, dairy and eggs, we become weak, emaciated, anaemic and ultimately die. I had failed to question whether or not this was even true, which it isn't. More broadly than that, most of us don't stop to reflect on what we do to animals; we simply carry on doing what we have always done. But by living this way, we fail to consider the most important question we should all ask ourselves: how do we morally justify our exploitation of animals?

IT'S A QUESTION OF MORALITY

There are so many reasons why veganism is the best choice. However, the fundamental argument, the one that underpins all others, is a question of morality – is eating animal products right or wrong? Any counterargument that you might hear needs to address this core point. But what do we mean by right or wrong? Well, moral philosophy is a thorny subject that has engaged some of the world's greatest thinkers, dating back to antiquity. It would be easy to get bogged down in theorising, but, for our purposes, it is sufficient to think about morality in terms of what most people would consider to be the values that we should live by and that we can all broadly agree on: respect, kindness, generosity and so on.

One of the core values of most relevance to any argument related to the consumption of animal products is that of cruelty – is it right or wrong to needlessly inflict pain and suffering on others? Only a deranged sociopath would disagree that being wilfully cruel is morally wrong, and although there may be some extreme exceptions to this rule (causing a murderous dictator to suffer so that millions of his subjects might be liberated obviously has utilitarian value and is objectively the right thing to do), these are outliers. Most of us can live by the maxim that we should try to avoid being cruel at all costs.

It is in this context of what is right and wrong according to our core values that any argument about animal exploitation needs to be judged. After all, veganism is an ethical stance against needless animal exploitation – it's not specifically about diet, although food is the primary reason why we use animals. Veganism is instead a social justice issue that recognises that non-human animals deserve autonomy, moral consideration and the recognition that their lives are far more valuable than the reasons we use to justify exploiting them. Although not everyone thinks about animal consumption from this ethical perspective, instead choosing to ignore the question, or framing it in terms of human nature or cultural norms, we can always bring it back to whether it is the right and moral thing to do.

Because issues of right and wrong are commonly shadowed by what is legal and illegal, it can be easy to presume that what we do to animals isn't that bad. After all, if it was so obviously wrong, surely it would be illegal. But does legality equal morality? Should something be accepted as ethical simply because it is allowed under law? We need only look to the past to recognise that legality does not equal morality. After all, apartheid was legal, slavery was legal, the Holocaust was legal, as were other acts of genocide that have taken place throughout history. If we were to subscribe to the belief that legality equals morality, then that would mean each country's legal system determines what is moral, but that is not how we determine what is right and wrong in an ethical sense.

THE CATALYST FOR CHANGE

Everything started to change for me in May 2014, when, at the age of 20, I was browsing through the news on the

BBC website and came across a piece about a truck carrying 6,000 chickens that had crashed on the way to a slaughter-house near Manchester. I clicked on the story and was horrified to read that many of the birds had died immediately on impact – in total, around 1,500. However, what disturbed me even more was the fact that thousands of the chickens had survived and were left lying on the side of the road, bleeding out with broken bones, combs, beaks and wings, mutilated and suffering. It was the first time I had ever found myself empathising with animals whom I consumed and thinking about our treatment of them from an ethical point of view. Consequently, I was forced to confront the fact that these animals have the capacity to suffer, something that, although obvious, I had never stopped to consider. It also occurred to me that they therefore had a preference to avoid that feeling of suffering. This led me to empathise not only with the chickens involved in that crash but also the chickens who were being farmed for me. They too, after all, suffered. Except, they were suffering because of the choices that I made.

At this point in my life, I was a self-proclaimed KFC addict. In fact, I visited my local KFC, which was only a ten-minute walk away, so often that the workers knew my name and my favourite order: a Zinger Box Meal, towered up. To say that I enjoyed KFC would be an understatement – I absolutely loved it. My bi-weekly trip to KFC not only provided me with a meal, it also formed a huge part of my identity and life at that time.

Like most people, I precariously balanced on the tightrope of mocking people who didn't want to hurt animals while simultaneously professing myself an animal lover. Yet in that moment, reading about the crash, I recognised the absurdity of my balancing act and gave myself an ultimatum: I could either bury my head in the sand, ignoring the feelings of guilt and discomfort that causing suffering to an animal created within me, or live by the new principles that I was beginning to form and change my lifestyle. I opted for the latter.

I had realised something important about myself. My values were not in alignment with my actions. I wasn't alone. As a society, we are overwhelmingly against animal cruelty. Most of us think that harming animals is reprehensible. But animals are subjected to violence every single day on farms and in slaughterhouses. So why are we selective in our compassion towards animals? And why are we only outraged by some forms of animal cruelty?

ANIMAL FARMING IS ANIMAL CRUELTY

If cruelty is defined as causing unnecessary and intentional physical or mental harm, what we do to animals must constitute acts of cruelty. We cut off their tails, we castrate them, we forcibly impregnate them, we take their babies away from them, we lock them in cages where they can't turn around. We load them into trucks and take them to slaughterhouses where we cut their throats or force them into gas chambers – and these are just the standard, legal practices. But perhaps even more insidious than that, we don't just ignore that these acts cause physical and mental harm, we go so far as to call them humane.

I often ask people to define what the word 'humane' means to them. Normally people respond by saying that it's the pursuit of reducing suffering for animals. If this is the case, then even by our subjective definition of the word, the most humane thing we can do for these animals is to not needlessly farm and kill them. This is the only way to extend the reduction of their suffering to its fullest extent.

But to work out whether or not what we do is objectively humane, and therefore right or wrong, we need only look at the literal definition of the word – having or showing compassion or benevolence – and apply synonyms for the word 'humane' to the acts we perform on them: is it 'benevolent' to mutilate piglets or to separate newborn babies from their mothers? Is it 'kind' to selectively breed chickens so that they cannot stand and their organs fail? And, most importantly, is it 'compassionate' to exploit and ultimately take the life of an animal who does not need or want to die? By any obvious standard, the answer to all of these questions is no. And regardless of the farming methods used, humane slaughter is an oxymoron, as it is impossible to take an animal's life needlessly and against their will in a compassionate, benevolent or kind way (there's more on this in chapter three). By any objective definition of these words, we would say these actions are not only inhumane, they are also acts of cruelty, which, as a society, as well as individuals, we are against and should therefore oppose and denounce. Yet we do not. We support and defend these industries, even though doing so contradicts our values.

People often call vegans extremists, and yet veganism is merely living by the principle that if I am against cruelty then I will do what I can to avoid perpetuating systems that cause physical and mental harm to animals. It is a clear indictment of how ingrained our state of cognitive dissonance is that we see attempts at moral consistency as signs of extremism. Is it not strange that we call those who kill dogs animal abusers, those who kill pigs normal and those who kill neither extremists? Is it not odd that someone who smashes a car window to rescue a dog on a hot day is viewed as a hero but someone who rescues a piglet suffering on a farm is a criminal?

THE ISSUE IS OUR MENTALITY

The story about the crash involving the chickens encouraged me to re-evaluate how I viewed animals and to challenge myself and reflect on my justifications for eating meat. As a result, I became vegetarian. Unfortunately, I was still not aware of what happens to dairy cows and egg-laying hens, nor did I grasp the full extent of how significantly animal exploitation has permeated our society. Truth be told, even as a vegetarian I thought vegans were too militant and extreme. However, that changed about seven months after the chicken truck crash when I watched a documentary called *Earthlings*.

The film uses undercover footage to expose what happens to animals in farms, slaughterhouses, research laboratories, puppy mills and other facilities where animals are exploited. It is relentlessly graphic and objective in its depiction of what happens to animals. At one point in the documentary, the narrator, Joaquin Phoenix, recites a quote from the nineteenth-century philosopher Ralph Waldo Emerson: 'You have just dined, and however scrupulously the slaughterhouse is concealed in the graceful distance of miles, there is complicity.' I felt angry and frustrated with myself as I acknowledged that even though I was vegetarian, I was still guilty of perpetuating these systems of violence that so utterly disgusted me. The animal products on my plate existed because I paid people, albeit indirectly, to cause suffering to animals. Just because the knife wasn't in my hand, or the blood on my clothes, I was still complicit – just as bloodstained, just as culpable.

After the film had finished, I went and sat with my pet hamster Rupert. He was my first real animal companion – aside from Batman, a black goldfish I had as a child – and the first animal I had ever formed a deep connection with. He was wonderful and brought such joy to my life. He was unbeliev-ably cute, and I would often give him treats just so I could sit and watch as he grasped the food with his tiny paws and pro-ceeded to nibble his way through whatever snack I had given him. So, to cheer myself up, I got him a small piece of broccoli – his favourite – and let him sit in my hands while he ate it.

As I watched him, I thought back to a part of the docu-mentary in which a guinea pig is being held up by a worker who is also injecting the helpless animal with some sort of undisclosed chemical. The clip is not as disturbing as the majority of the scenes shown, many of which are exception-ally brutal. However, the similarities between Rupert and the guinea pig caused me to think of Rupert being experimented on, and the fear in the guinea pig's eyes reminded me of the fear I had on occasion seen in Rupert's eyes. One time when he had been running around on the sofa, he had peered too far over the edge and fallen off, landing awkwardly on one of his legs. He'd let out a shrill noise and begun to limp around frantically. He'd looked so scared and confused.

I thought about Rupert's distress and how an animal's capacity to feel pain is much the same as my own. I also thought about his personality and the fact that he had likes and dislikes. For instance, he loved the broccoli he was eating right at that moment, but he didn't really like kale. He was also an exceptionally lazy hamster, reluctant to apply himself to anything that required significant physical exertion. He wasn't keen on his running wheel, so I'd got him a running ball instead. But every time I placed him in it, he would walk around for a few minutes and then stop and take out the food he had been storing in his cheeks and eat that instead. Once he had finished eating, he would then proceed to curl up and go to sleep. In the end, I gave him free rein of the room, taking him out of his home and placing him on the floor so he could potter about and do as he pleased.

As I continued to watch Rupert eat his piece of broccoli, I thought about all the animals who were exploited on my behalf but who had personalities just like Rupert. Who had likes and dislikes, and who experienced fear and pain, joy and happiness. The ability of animals to have these subjective experiences was outlined in the European Union's 2007 Treaty of Lisbon, which determined that animals are sentient beings. In 2021, the UK government also announced a law that would formally recognise the sentience of animals (including farmed animals).

But even outside of these declarations, animals have been documented as showing emotions, including empathy, such as in a study where a rat was placed in water and another rat had the option to either pull a lever that saved the one in the water or pull a lever that released a chocolate treat. The rats pulled the lever to save the rat in distress, even though it meant forgoing the treat. When there was no other rat to save, they would just go for the lever that gave them the treat. Interestingly, if the rat with the choice of levers had been placed in the water previously and had gone through that experience, they were quicker to help the rat they had the chance to save.[1] This study showed that rats display pro-social behaviour and exhibit empathy, even in situations where doing so comes at a disadvantage to them.

There was also a study carried out in which researchers housed sixteen groups of six pigs. Two of the pigs from each group were taken to be trained, with one thinking that something good would happen when a piece of music was played and the other that something bad was going to happen. They then placed one of the trained pigs back into the pen with the pigs that didn't have any association with the music. The researchers found that the untrained pigs would show emotional contagion, reacting to the behaviour of the pig who was expecting something bad to happen by exhibiting signs of stress.[2]

While the findings of these studies may shed light on the complexity of non-human animals, the studies themselves are undeniably cruel. By referencing them, I am not condoning the studies, which were undertaken to satisfy human curiosity, not to help animals. After all, rats and pigs shouldn't need to display empathy to warrant not being needlessly exploited, although, sadly, even the fact that they do hasn't made a difference anyway.

It is ironic that we often believe that empathy and complex emotions only really exist in humans but we then fail to empathise with the animals who suffer at our hands. Primatologist Frans de Waal refers to the denial of these emotions and capabilities in non-human animals as 'anthropodenial',[3] a term he coined to describe the behaviour of discounting the complexity of other animals. As he states, 'Anyone who wants to make the case that a tickled ape, who almost chokes on his hoarse giggles, must be in a different state of mind from a tickled child has his work cut out for him.'[4]

But this denial of an animal's intelligence is one of the main defences we have to justify what we do to them, as studies have shown that people find it more morally wrong to eat animals who are characterised as being 'mindful', with there being a strong negative correlation between people's perceived intelligence of an animal and the animal's edibility.[5] By believing that humans are exceptional, it's easier for us to deny the animality of humans but also the humanity of non-human animals, and if we were to challenge the idea of what we classify as being human-only traits, it would fundamentally challenge the way we treat and interact with other animals.

And so as I watched Rupert eating, I thought of all the other animals incarcerated in farms, cages and slaughterhouses, their autonomy denied to them, their bodies reduced to nothing other than commodities, objects whose personalities we disregard and whose lives we treat with such contempt. I thought of someone trying to hurt Rupert and how that would make me feel. What right did I have to inflict pain and suffering on other living beings, especially ones with the characteristics and traits that I held in such high regard where Rupert was concerned?

I then considered how I had bought Rupert for ten pounds – this was the value that his existence had been assigned. Such a small sum. By purchasing Rupert, I had treated him as a commodity and yet in my eyes he wasn't an object over which an exchange of money could constitute ownership. But if Rupert wasn't a commodity, then why should any other animal be? Why should any other animal have their autonomy denied them?

It was at this point that I realised being vegetarian wasn't enough. I saw that the issue of animal exploitation far transcends the purchasing of meat and is instead fundamentally an issue of how we view our relationship with other sentient life. Consumption is only a symptom. The real problem is our mentality, a mentality that judges some lives to be less important because of the pleasure we get from consuming their flesh or wearing their skin. We have allowed our physical and intellectual capabilities to make us tyrants over every other species on this planet. I have heard it said before that to the animals we are the devils of this planet and this world is their hell, a place of subjugation and pain. I can't see any rational reason why this isn't the case.

THE MORAL DIFFERENCE BETWEEN A BROCCOLI STALK AND A PIG'S THROAT

Those who argue in favour of eating animals will often say that because animals are less intelligent, lack the cognitive capabilities of humans and are unable to display the same level of agency and responsibility or engage in social contracts, it is therefore morally acceptable to exploit them. However, do we actually believe that intelligence should define worth of life or that being more intelligent than someone else gives you the right to harm and exploit them? Disturbingly, this line of thinking could also then be used to justify harming human infants and those who are cognitively impaired, because they also lack these abilities. Thankfully, not only do we still think such people deserve moral consideration, we often give them special consideration because of their lower cognition and agency. The fact that we simultaneously justify giving animals less consideration for the same reasons is yet another example of how inconsistently we apply our moral framework.

Even if we truly lived by the philosophy that intelligence defines worth of life, we wouldn't farm the animals that we do. For example, pigs have been shown to be at least as intelligent as dogs, if not more so. Yet we love one species, welcoming them into our homes, giving them names and feeling grief when they die, while we staple numbered tags through the ears of the other, treating them as objects and then paying for and disregarding their deaths. Many people even go so far as to mock those who mourn the deaths of farm animals. One species we turn into ashes so we can remember and cherish their life, the other we turn into faeces. Besides, if we truly did believe that intelligence defines worth of life, we would all be vegan, as the plants we consume are quantifiably less intelligent than the animals we eat.

That being said, some people make the claim that eating plants is morally the same as eating animals, as both are living organisms. However, while plants are alive and capable of doing some amazing things, their intelligence does not equal sentience, nor does it mean that they have subjective

21

experiences and can feel pain. A plant lacks a central nervous system, a brain and pain receptors. So while animals respond to situations, plants instead react. This is why a Venus flytrap does not just close around flies but will close around anything that triggers the pressure stimuli on its trap. Animals, on the other hand, consciously respond to the situations they are in, which is why they won't just eat something because you try to feed it to them.

And besides, because of the feed used for animals and the fact that animal farming is the number one cause of rainforest deforestation[6] and habitat loss,[7] more plants are killed in the production of non-vegan foods than they are vegan foods. So, even if we did believe that plants suffer or that they deserve moral consideration due to being alive, we would still be morally obliged to be vegan anyway. Ultimately, people who say that it's hypocritical to eat plants but not animals are trying to convince themselves that there is no discernible moral difference between chopping a broccoli stalk and cutting a pig's throat.

ARE OUR TASTEBUDS WORTH MORE THAN THEIR LIVES?

With the scale and severity of the violence we perpetuate against animals, you might presume our reason for doing so must be predicated on some deeply regrettable yet intrinsically necessary act for our survival. Yet once we have recognised that we don't need to consume animal products to be healthy, the primary reason for why we continue to do so is because we like eating them. We enjoy the taste of steak, bacon and cheese, and that fact alone is arguably the most persuasive explanation for our treatment of animals.

Even if many of us don't realise it, by placing taste at the heart of our justification for eating animal products, we are essentially saying that our pleasure is more important than any moral consideration. I can think of many situations in which an oppressor feels sensory pleasure at the expense of a victim, but those actions are in no way made more acceptable simply because of this. So why would the fact that we enjoy the taste of these products make what we do to animals justified as a result?

I think it is unlikely that any of us actually believe that sensory pleasure should be held up as a standard by which our actions are judged to be moral. This would be the equivalent of arguing that our tastebuds are worth more than the life and subjective experiences of a sentient being. But the reality is that when we eat any of these products, including dairy and eggs, an animal has either already been killed to produce it or is in the process of being exploited and will eventually be killed, and there is no moral justification that would make this prioritisation of taste over life acceptable. The fact that our enjoyment of these products only lasts for 15 minutes or so, the length of time it takes us to eat a meal, only further trivialises the idea of sensory pleasure being a moral justifier. It's unconscionable that billions of sentient beings have their lives filled with suffering and forcibly taken from them just for fleeting moments of pleasure. Lives obliterated for meals we eat and then forget about.

This argument becomes even more unreasonable when we consider that there are already so many great plant-based substitutes and foods available, including burgers, sausages, ice cream, milk, chocolate and even cheese (yes, there are good vegan ones, I promise). For nearly every animal product we previously enjoyed, we don't even have to give up the taste because there is an ever-growing range of delicious alternatives available.

IT'S NOT OUR DIFFERENCES THAT MATTER

At the centre of the moral justifications we use to defend animal consumption is the notion of 'speciesism', a term coined in 1970 by Richard Ryder, an ex-vivisectionist turned animal rights advocate. The term was then popularised in 1975 by the philosopher Peter Singer in his book *Animal Liberation*. Singer defines speciesism as being 'a prejudice or attitude of bias in favour of the interests of members of one's own species and against those of members of other species'. In other words, a prejudice that says it's OK to favour a human's desire to eat a bacon sandwich over a pig's desire to not be killed in a gas chamber.

Favouring one's own species in a situation where you had to choose between saving a member of your own species or a different one – for example, choosing to save a human child over a dog from a fire – could, of course, be morally justified. But this doesn't justify speciesism or arbitrarily causing harm to non-human animals. In the same way, faced with an unavoidable decision between allowing a young child or a 95-year-old human to live, favouring the child in this circumstance does not justify ageism or allowing the elderly to suffer or die needlessly.

One of the main issues with a speciesist mentality is that it creates arbitrary distinctions between different species of animals, such as between dogs and pigs. Even more importantly, it creates a mindset of discrimination that in turn can facilitate exploitation. It carries the idea of human superiority to the extreme, to the point that trivial and needless human desires are morally permissible, such as skinning animals for a fur or leather jacket, forcing animals into slaughterhouses for a sandwich, or separating newborn calves from their mothers so that we can drink their mothers' milk.

It is important to note that anti-speciesists recognise that humans and non-humans are vastly different in many ways, including our physical forms, intelligence and sociability, among other things. However, it is not the differences that are relevant when deciding whether non-humans matter morally but instead the similarities – most fundamentally sentience, meaning the capacity to feel and experience subjectively. If it is sentience that makes human animals worthy of moral consideration then it is sentience that makes non-human animals worthy of moral consideration too.

Even if we were to believe that there is a moral distinction between a human and a non-human, that distinction is surely not so significant that it justifies the unnecessary torture and slaughter of hundreds of billions of animals every single year. In fact, any amount of moral value should prohibit the act of slaughter, and the objective reality that animals can suffer and have subjective experiences immediately withdraws any notion of acceptability when it comes to exploiting them.

However, speciesism is so ingrained and normalised within society that we don't even consider it a problem. Many humans view non-human animals with such little regard that the very concept of animals deserving moral consideration is seen as offensive, as they believe that recognising that other animals also deserve basic rights is somehow demeaning to our own species. People will often laugh at those who raise these issues, but of course it's much easier to mock the idea of animals having basic rights than it is to look at a piece of steak on a dinner plate and attempt to justify why animals have such little worth that they should have their throats cut simply because we enjoy eating a piece of their body.

Ultimately, it's important for us to recognise that we have moral agency and are able to rationalise and scrutinise our decisions. Instead of killing animals being a prerequisite for survival, as is the case for certain species of wild animals, we can (and should) hold ourselves accountable when making decisions that pertain to what is right and wrong.

Some people believe that to be vegan means you have to be an animal lover or be someone who goes out of their way to be kind to animals. But it's not an act of kindness to not needlessly hurt someone. If we walk down the street and don't kick a dog, that's not an act of kindness. In the same way, avoiding forcing animals into gas chambers and macerators and onto kill lines isn't an act of benevolence – it's an act of justice and respect for the basic moral consideration that all animals deserve.

2.

OUR PAST SHOWS US WHY VEGANISM MUST BE OUR FUTURE

When I have conversations with people about veganism, they often say, 'I agree with you, which is why I try to buy meat from small local family farms when I can.' However, the idea that a farm being nearby means that it's more ethical clearly doesn't hold up when you consider that every farm is local to someone. Plus, 98 per cent of farms in the USA are classed as 'family farms',[1] which makes you realise that the notion of a family farm has nothing to do with an animal's wellbeing but is instead a marketing ploy to make us think of a romanticised ideal of farming that simply doesn't exist.

However, I used to have this attitude too. One of the biggest misconceptions about veganism is that it exists to oppose factory farming and that the moral concerns around eating animal products are purely focused on these intensive practices. This is one way in which we can avoid dealing with the morality of animal consumption: we perceive factory farming to be the problem, not the mindset that has allowed factory farming to exist in the first place. But by looking at our past, we can see that factory farming was not the beginning of the problem and why our future needs to be progressive and not regressive. So how did we get to where we are today?

We often romanticise the history of animal farming and talk about a return to 'idyllic' days gone by. However, while this perception acknowledges how destructive and cruel animal farming has become, it unfortunately overlooks the fact that it has never been idyllic or indeed humane. In fact, our history of animal exploitation is fraught with examples of why idealising the past won't help us to address the fundamental problems with farming today. It is also indicative of the deep misconceptions people have when it comes to the mass production of animals for human consumption.

PERCEPTION VERSUS REALITY

I am always amazed by how many people, when asked, say that they are opposed to the mistreatment of animals. For example, a poll conducted in the USA in 2017 showed that 49 per cent of Americans agreed with the statement 'I support a ban on the factory farming of animals', with 47 per cent even supporting a ban on slaughterhouses.[2] What's even more striking, though, is that 58 per cent of people also believed that farmed animals are treated well. This ultimately shows how disconnected we are from the process of what happens to animals and how uninformed we are; 50 per cent of respondents were against a method of farming that produces more than 99 per cent of the animal products in the USA, according to government census data, yet the majority of people also simultaneously believed that farmed animals are treated well. There's a clear contradiction between what consumers want, what they are actually buying and what they think they are buying.

So how is it that an industry that half of the population wants banned is not only the most dominant system of animal-product production but also goes almost entirely unopposed and is even perpetuated by the people who say they are against it?

In politics, there is a concept called the Overton window, which is sometimes referred to as 'the window of discourse'. It is defined as the range of ideas that the general public is willing to consider and may accept at any given time. So, from a politician's perspective, it contains the policies that the majority of voters see as reasonable and legitimate. The window will shift over time, both for better and worse, due to social factors and changing perceptions. Campaigners seek to actively move it by persuading people of the value of ideas that they may have first found extreme. For example, women's right to vote was once an extreme concept to many that ultimately became a social norm.

This idea of an ever-shifting window of what we perceive as acceptable can be applied to the evolution of animal exploitation as well, as the system and the scale of what we have today came about through incremental changes over a long period of time. Unfortunately, these changes have been defined by increasing industrialisation and aspirations of further efficiency and profitability. We have made farms more intensive, confining more animals in smaller spaces, while also breeding them to grow bigger, faster. If we look at factory farming in particular, the advent of industrialised animal farming started in the 1920s but became increasingly significant from the 1960s onwards, and we have seen the scale continue to increase ever since. However, to understand how we have created the system of agriculture that we have today, we need to go way back to the time before we even had an agricultural system at all.

FROM HUMBLE BEGINNINGS

Early humans were nomadic beings who relied on hunting and gathering for survival. In practice, this means that for most of our history we were opportunistic scavengers who primarily ate plants, insects, some small animals and carrion. In fact, it is believed that early humans may have often resorted to eating bone marrow from bigger animals, as we were unable to compete with larger, stronger predators and had to consequently wait for them to finish eating the animals that they had killed. By the time it was our turn, there wouldn't be anything particularly substantial left, except of course the bones, from which we could then extract the marrow. As a result, for most of our existence, humans were very much in the middle of the food chain, able to hunt smaller animals but still at the mercy of predators.

Despite animals making up only a portion of the prehistoric diet, people who are anti-vegan often argue that our brains developed as a consequence of us hunting and eating meat. However, we don't know for certain why our brains began to grow and develop in the way that they did, and there are other theories as well: for example, that the consumption of foods such as potatoes was actually responsible for the growth of our brains. In many ways, this appears to make more sense. Because our brains use around 20 to 25 per cent of all our energy, and because the body's main source of energy is glucose, consuming foods high in carbohydrates would have been highly beneficial for our cognitive development. The argument becomes even more compelling when you consider that the use of fire is often believed to have contributed to our brains growing bigger. Fire allowed us to cook foods that would have previously been hard to digest, such as wild grains and tubers, which became staples in our diet and are some of the most carbohydrate-dense foods on the planet.

This theory was further supported by a study published in 2021 that was carried out by an international research team.[3] The researchers analysed the fossilised dental plaque of early humans and found oral bacteria specifically adapted to break down starch, which would have only existed if starch was a regular part of their diet.[4]

Of course, it is true that the cooking of food aided the consumption of meat as well, making it safer and easier to digest. But even if we believe that eating meat did contribute to *Homo sapiens'* 'Cognitive Revolution', the name often given to the period when our brains developed, it would still be illogical to attempt to justify the consumption of animals for this reason, especially as we can hardly make the argument that eating cooked meat is now making us a more intelligent society. Whatever happened tens of thousands of years ago, however significant it was, should have no bearing on determining whether or not what we do to animals is justified now.

As a consequence of the Cognitive Revolution, we began to colonise the world. Starting in Africa, where *Homo sapiens* originated from, we migrated to different parts of the planet, where unfortunately a pattern emerged: the demise of the world's megafauna. We colonised Australia, where we encountered animals such as flightless birds twice the size of ostriches, marsupial lions, giant koalas and diprotodons – huge wombats weighing around two and a half tons. Unfortunately, out of the 24 Australian animal species that weighed more than 50 kilograms, 23 became extinct.

It was a similar story when the first *Homo sapiens* made it to the Americas, travelling from Alaska into Canada and then the USA, where we encountered mammoths, sabretooth cats, six-metre-high giant ground sloths and huge rodents the size of bears, before heading into Central and South America, where we came across all kinds of reptiles and birds. Sadly, 50 out of the 60 genera of large animals that existed in South America went extinct, as did 34 out of the 47 genera in North America. These were species and genera that had existed for tens of millions of years, surviving changing climates, but they were no match for humans, who wiped out hundreds of millions of years' worth of evolution.

THE DAWN OF AGRICULTURE

During this time of colonisation, we entered the Neolithic period, which started around 12,000 years ago. It was at this time that we discovered we could grow some plants from seeds and domesticate certain species of animals. Consequently, we started what has come to be known as the 'Agricultural Revolution'. Agriculture first began in the Fertile Crescent, an area of land that spans the Middle East and includes modern-day Iraq, Syria and Egypt, among others. It was highly fertile due to irrigation from the large rivers in the region and the diverse climate.

As a result of agriculture, we stopped being nomadic beings and began to live more sedentary and settled lives. Our population also began to grow considerably. There were only an estimated 4 million humans on the planet 12,000 years ago;[5] agriculture has allowed for the global population to reach almost 8 billion people and counting.

It was during the Agricultural Revolution that the animals we now farm by the billion were first domesticated and we began to use them for their meat, secretions, skin and labour. This process required animals to be turned into subjugated beings, with their desires and natural instincts removed as much as possible. As a result, animals were whipped, bridled, leashed and mutilated, with male animals often being castrated if they weren't being used for breeding. Many of these practices that were carried out on animals thousands of years ago are still routine today.

Take dairy production, for example. Throughout history, farmers have killed male calves shortly after their birth, as is still commonplace in many dairy farms today. Ancient farmers would alternatively tie rings of thorns around the mouths of the calves so that it hurt their mothers if they tried to suckle. Farmers around the world currently use devices that are designed to perform the same purpose. Other farmers would kill the offspring, eat them and then stuff the skin, smearing it with the mother's urine to trick her into producing more milk that humans could then consume. Disturbingly, this practice can still be seen today, with some farmers stuffing dead calves with hay to try to trick mother cows into producing more milk. A similar practice is known as 'grafting', whereby a farmer skins a dead calf and places it over the body of another calf to trick the mother of the dead animal into thinking that the other baby is her own.

Many of us believe that farming only became cruel when we started factory farming in the twentieth century; however, it is clear that as soon as we started to farm animals, we began to abuse them, with many of the practices we now find abhorrent having existed since the domestication of animals began. It was our ancestors who started us on the road to the animal-agriculture industries of the twentieth and twenty-first centuries. In many ways, the fact that animal farming has such violent origins makes it easier to understand how farmers were able to keep pushing the boundaries of what would be considered acceptable, shifting bit by bit the Overton window of animal farming.

THE CHICKEN OF TOMORROW

The Industrial Revolution in the eighteenth and nineteenth centuries facilitated the next significant progression in our agriculture development, especially in relation to selective breeding. The practice of selectively choosing to breed specific animals together based on them having desirable traits is a manufactured version of natural selection; however, instead of animals evolving for reasons advantageous to them, animals are changed by humans for reasons advantageous to us.

Selective breeding has been around for thousands of years, particularly in the case of dogs. However, the Industrial Revolution saw it becoming established as a scientific practice and led to breeding programmes for sheep, who were bred to grow larger quantities of wool, and for cattle, who were bred to grow larger in size and be more profitable for cattle farmers. In the case of sheep, because farmers found those that shed the least amount of wool to be the most desirable and easiest to profit from, over time they continued to selectively breed the animals to the point that they no longer naturally shed their wool, as they had done for millennia. This is why sheep now have to be sheared.

Other animals that have been selectively bred include dairy cows, who produce significantly more milk than their offspring would have drunk; pigs, who have been selectively bred to grow larger; and egg-laying hens, who can now produce up to 300 eggs a year, which is significantly higher than the 10 to 15 eggs their presumed wild ancestor, the red jungle fowl, lays.

Chickens raised for their meat, referred to as broiler chickens, have also been selectively bred. In fact, in the late 1940s there was a United States Department of Agriculture (USDA)-

organised 'Chicken of Tomorrow' contest, the purpose of which was to breed a chicken with larger breasts and legs that would make chicken meat more cost effective and desirable for consumers. After the winner of the contest was announced, there was even a celebratory parade with floats depicting the poultry industry, which rather bizarrely included a woman who had been crowned the festival 'Broiler Queen' perched on top of a car waving. Is there not something very odd about the idea of crowning someone queen of broiler chickens? For the chickens, the contest was anything but a cause for celebration; it was the start of a significant increase in the number of them who would be made to suffer and then be killed.

The selective breeding of broilers continued to the point that they are today bred to reach slaughter age in only six weeks, a rate of growth 300 per cent faster than in 1960. In that time, they reach a weight four times heavier on average than chickens raised in 1957. Chickens have suffered hugely as a consequence of this selective breeding, with many of them dying from organ failure, suffering from immune system problems and being unable to move due to their excessive weight, meaning they are unable to reach food and water points.

We often make appeals to nature to justify our consumption of animals. But even if we believe that eating animals is a natural part of being human, and overlook the point that what is natural is not always what is best, morally or otherwise, what we do to animals is about as far removed from nature as possible. It is a wholly industrialised process that involves selective breeding, artificial insemination and mutilations, to name but a few of the terrible practices that happen every day. It treats animals as if they are simply replaceable objects, commodities who have no value beyond the price tag on the supermarket shelf.

THE DIRTY MILK CRISIS

As well as selective breeding, the Industrial Revolution also saw a huge rise in milk and dairy consumption. Although milk had been consumed for thousands of years, in rural communities it was a localised, cottage industry with a dairy farm supplying the immediate community. However, during this period of time, people began leaving their subsistence farms for large towns and cities, creating an opportunity for the dairy industry to become increasingly professionalised. This urbanisation also meant that milk now had to travel greater distances to reach people, which posed a specific problem for dairy farmers. Dry foods and grains could be transported easily, and even meat could be dried or salted, but at the time there was no way of preserving milk in its raw form.

Milk is an ideal environment for bacteria, making things even more difficult for the dairy industry. Diseases such as bovine tuberculosis could contaminate milk, killing many people, particularly children. In Britain alone, an estimated 500,000 infant deaths between 1850 and 1950 were caused by tuberculosis-infected milk, and as many as 30 per cent of all tuberculosis deaths before 1930 are thought to have originated from milk.[6] There was also the risk of milk being contaminated with scarlet fever, diphtheria and typhoid. In fact, it got so bad that in the 1850s a New York journalist demanded to know why the police weren't investigating dairy farmers as milk was so risky to consume. By the 1880s, analyses of milk samples in New Jersey found liquifying colonies of bacteria to be so high in number that they were unable to count them. These problems were compounded even further during the summer months, when milk would go off much quicker. As a result, a common gastrointestinal condition referred to as 'summer complaint' due to it appearing in the warmer months is strongly believed to have come from milk.

There were other issues plaguing the dairy industry at that time, including a distrust of dairy farmers that had built up due to the multitude of substances they were adding to their products. For example, in an attempt to make more money, dairy producers would thin their milk by adding water and then use chalk, plaster dust or dyes to recolour the liquid. An article published in the *Indianapolis News* in 1900 reported that a family discovered a pint of milk they had bought was wriggling due to the fact there were worms inside the stagnant water that the farmer had used to thin it. It was also reported that farmers were adding a layer of pureed calf brains to milk to give it the appearance of having a rich cream.

More disturbing still, without refrigeration or effective preserving methods, farmers began to add formaldehyde to their milk. This was done as a reaction to how contaminated it was, as it was believed the chemical could help kill the bacteria. By the 1890s, formaldehyde use had become so widespread that the terms 'embalmed milk' and 'embalmed meat' were used to describe the practice. As you might expect, the preservative made people sick – in 1899 alone, 400 children died in Indiana after drinking embalmed milk.[7] Thankfully, dairy producers began to be prosecuted for using formaldehyde. The practice was banned in the USA in 1906, while in the UK formaldehyde was legal for use in milk up until 1912, as was borax, a compound that is used in cleaning products to get rid of mould and mildew.[8] The dirty milk crisis was so serious that increasing milk sanitation is viewed as one of the main reasons why infant mortality in the USA dropped so significantly in the early twentieth century.

However, during the dirty milk crisis, despite the risks, the product was increasingly being marketed as an important food for children. Medical professionals worried that the urbanisation of families could place a strain on mothers and jeopardise the quality of their breast milk or even lead to them not being able to produce any at all. This encouragement to drink cow's milk proved not only to be incredibly dangerous for infants, who were being exposed to bacteria and chemicals from the milk, but it was also significant in shaping our perceived idea that cow's milk is important for children.

THE UNDERGROUND CHEESE BUNKERS

Alongside pasteurisation, which became widespread in the 1920s, the turmoil of the early twentieth century also changed our relationship with milk for ever. During the First World War, governments sent powdered and tinned milk overseas for the Allied troops. Due to this, significantly higher quantities of milk needed to be produced, and many farmers consequently began to grow their dairy herds, breeding more animals into existence or turning their diversified farms into solely dairy farms. After the war ended, the demand for dairy products dropped dramatically but the supply of milk remained just as high. This led to low prices and dairy farmers unionising to demand a higher price for their milk. However, instead of encouraging a reduction in the production of milk, the government worked to increase the amount being consumed by perpetuating the idea that milk is important and necessary for human health and development. This included federally subsidised milk advertising and the introduction of school milk programmes, as well as USDA guidance that children should be consuming four glasses of milk a day.

When the Second World War started, a similar supply chain was set up to provide troops with long-life dairy products. Once again, there was a drop-off in demand after the war had ended. This led to the US government creating a buy-back scheme called the Milk Price Support Program, in which they would purchase surplus storable dairy products, such as butter and cheese, from farmers. This scheme did nothing to address the oversupply of dairy products and instead encouraged it, as farmers knew they would get a constant price for the dairy they produced.

The problem became so prevalent that the US government began to store the huge surplus of dairy products in vast warehouses, having spent billions of dollars of taxpayers' money to buy them from the producers in the first place. This eventually led to the creation of so-called 'government cheese'. Under pressure due to the billions of dollars the government was spending, in 1981 Ronald Reagan began to give some of the surplus processed cheese to people in need.

To this day, the US government still buys back dairy products, with the USDA purchasing $50 million of surplus milk in 2018. There is so much surplus cheese being stored by the US government that it is estimated it would be as big as the US Capitol building if it was formed into one giant wheel. Even more alarming, it is estimated that between 2017 and 2018 the amount of surplus cheese grew by 6 per cent, while at the same time per capita milk consumption declined, suggesting that instead of adapting to the changing market, the industry is instead continuing to rely on the taxpayer to subsidise the difference.

It was a similar story in the EU as well, with the Common Agricultural Policy, set up during the second half of the twentieth century, guaranteeing farmers a minimum price for what they produced no matter how much they produced. The policy was created to increase Europe's food sufficiency and security following the Second World War, as well as providing a stable income for those working in agriculture.

However, it also created huge agricultural surpluses, leading to the creation of so-called butter and beef mountains and milk lakes. It is bad enough that production of dairy involves so much exploitation and suffering for animals, but there is something inherently wrong with a system that uses taxpayer funds to knowingly and needlessly overproduce, resulting in masses of milk and other dairy products that will never even be consumed.

UNDERMINING THE MIRACLES OF MODERN MEDICINE

The biggest catalyst in the creation of modern-day farming has been the significant scientific and technological breakthroughs that have occurred since the Industrial Revolution. One of the most notable of these was the discovery of penicillin by Alexander Fleming in 1928, which led to the introduction of antibiotics, often referred to as the miracle of modern medicine. For the first time, common life-threatening infections could be treated and illnesses that were previously lethal became not only manageable but of little concern. The same was also true for illnesses that affected farm animals.

The other most significant breakthrough came from Louis Pasteur, who initially developed vaccines for anthrax and chicken cholera in the late nineteenth century. In the twentieth century, we eradicated smallpox and greatly reduced the prevalence of polio, measles, diphtheria and tetanus, among others, through the use of vaccination. Vaccines also began to be extensively used on farm animals to protect them from diseases such as cattle plague, rotavirus and infectious bronchitis.

The discovery of antibiotics and vaccines came at the same time as a rise in a deeper understanding of animal behaviour, alongside increasing awareness of vitamins and animal nutrition. For the first time, we were able to work out exactly what animals needed to survive and not have to worry about diseases killing them off if they were to be farmed inside in larger numbers, where unhygienic conditions combined with overcrowding would otherwise make farming unviable. Bringing animals inside gave the farmers much more control of the process, allowing them to raise more animals using less space and resources. It also meant they could control the feed, temperature and lighting, which allowed them to optimise the growth of the animals further.

THE RISE OF FACTORY FARMING

The first animals to be farmed intensively were chickens, in the 1920s and 30s, with vitamin D supplementation allowing chicken farmers to raise the animals in confinement all year round, as they no longer needed sunlight to thrive. A more commercially oriented poultry sector emerged alongside the creation of early model battery cages. At this time, chicken meat was mainly seen as a by-product of the egg industry, meaning that cockerels were viewed as less desirable. Chicken farmers would castrate the male chickens by cutting the testes out of the birds in order to make their breasts bigger and therefore more profitable.

The era of factory farming is widely regarded as having started in Britain not long after the Second World War in 1947. It was brought about by the introduction of a new subsidy in the Agriculture Act that incentivised farmers to produce more food, improve breeding, maximise animal management and incorporate new technology into agriculture. The motivation was to increase the self-sufficiency of food production in the UK and decrease reliance on imported meat. In essence, similar to the Common Agricultural Policy, it was seen as a way of increasing food security in the wake of a world war and food rationing.

The end of the Second World War also brought about the rise of synthetic nitrogen fertilisers. Throughout the war, countries had built large-scale nitrate factories to produce bombs and the industry was simply able to transition these factories into the production of nitrate fertilisers instead. This allowed farmers to produce significantly larger amounts of feed for animals, meaning that not only could more animals be produced but there was less need for these animals to have access to outside areas, as they no longer needed to forage or graze for food.

Throughout the 1950s and 60s, the price of eggs and chicken meat began to plummet, causing smaller-scale producers to go bankrupt and be replaced by larger industrial operations, further compounding the problem. In fact, it was estimated that egg prices decreased so significantly in the 1950s that farmers had to triple the number of hens they kept to cover the price of the drop, leading to more hens being housed in confined spaces.

Then, in the mid 1960s, following on from the success of the poultry industry, the factory farming of pigs and cattle began, with farmers bringing the animals permanently indoors and relying heavily on antibiotics and feed to maximise their production. It was at this point that animal farming really began to take the shape that we recognise now, with the problem growing substantially into the 1980s, at which point huge meat-producing companies saw massive growth and market domination.

Many of these corporations expanded by recruiting small farms and contracting them to breed and produce animals. In this model, the animals are legally owned by the corporations, so the more farms that join, the more animals the companies own. This in turn leads to a higher supply of animals as the corporations force the farmers to adapt to their more intensive practices and scale up to meet the demands of the contracts, which then causes the prices to drop. This cycle makes it exceptionally difficult for independent farmers to compete with the corporations, and so more and more contract themselves out to the major corporations to survive, further perpetuating the problem. In fact, it is estimated that around 97 per cent of chicken farmers in the USA are currently contractors for these huge corporations.[9]

It's a similar story in UK, with companies such as Moy Park, who have a near monopoly on farmers in Northern Ireland, and Avara Foods contracting smaller farms to supply them with their animals. All of this leads to a lack of competition and a proverbial race to the bottom, where deregulation, lack of oversight and a monopolisation of the market creates declining standards for the humans and animals exploited within the industry.

This move to factory farming, coupled with the fact that consumers, by and large, have become used to being able to buy cheap meat, dairy and eggs, creates a self-fulfilling cycle that is killing trillions of animals, creating widespread chronic disease, destroying our environment, increasing the risk of pandemics and wasting trillions of dollars of taxpayers' money in the form of subsidies and bailouts.

To emphasise the power these corporations have, we need look no further than JBS, the biggest of all meatpackers. As reported by the Bureau of Investigative Journalism, they have an annual turnover of $50 billion and slaughter nearly 14 million animals every single day. They have also been found to have bought meat from a farm that was under investigation by Brazilian prosecutors for using modern-day human slaves (JBS said they stopped as soon as they were aware), faced allegations of buying cattle from ranches located on illegally deforested land (they say they planned to work on their supply chains), defended allegations of insider trading and admitted bribing politicians.[10] Yet, despite all of this, their products can still be found on the shelves of major supermarkets in the USA, Australia and the UK.

The industrialisation of farming is not restricted to the West. Since the 1990s, there has been a huge expansion of animal farming across Asia, particularly in China. In 1990, the country was the world's twenty-fourth largest producer of milk, but by 2017 it was the fourth biggest, behind only the EU, the USA and India. Likewise, in the 1980s, beef was known as 'millionaire's meat' in China; however, the country is now one of the biggest producers and consumers of beef. Overall, Chinese citizens are eating four times as much meat per year now than they did in the 1980s. Unfortunately, this trend is only going to increase as the industrialisation of animal farming continues to grow across not only China but the rest of Asia as well.

An ever-growing population currently means an ever-growing supply of animal products. Even in places such as the UK, where veganism is on the rise, there has been an alarming trend in the increasing number of so called 'mega-farms'. In fact, there was a 26 per cent increase in intensive factory farming in the UK between 2011 and 2017. US-style cattle feedlots, which are essentially confined grassless pens in which cattle are fattened up on grain for slaughter, have begun to be used in the UK as well.[11]

A GRIM FUTURE AWAITS US IF WE DON'T CHANGE DIRECTION

As we look towards the future, as well as the continuing selective breeding of animals and the growth of intensive farming, there have been several other disturbing ideas suggested as potential ways to feed a growing global population. One such idea put forward during a project to find sustainable solutions to UK animal farming involved removing the cerebral cortex of chickens and essentially lobotomising them and hooking them up to life-support machines to keep them alive. This really summarises just how far we have gone in devaluing the lives of non-human animals, to the point where lobotomising them is viewed as a potential way of making animal farming more sustainable, rather than no longer eating the animals in the first place.

Gene editing is another idea under discussion, with the USDA and the animal agriculture industries looking to control this new technology and find ways to incorporate it into factory farming. This could involve animals' genes being edited so that they are hornless or, more disturbingly, designing them to be blind or deaf so that they would be less distressed about being in crowded conditions.

Unfortunately, our history of animal mistreatment has created the industrial system of farming we have today, but instead of looking to our past to justify continuing down the same road, we should instead recognise the process that is going on right before our eyes and stop it now. We should in no way romanticise the farming of our past. While the industrialisation of animal agriculture has brought about disastrous consequences, there has never been a point in our farming history when animals were treated well. Small, local, family farms still operate by exploiting animals, and much of what happens to animals today is a result of practices that started long before factory farming existed.

The reality is, we have a broken relationship with animals. We have created a mindset that views other animals as subjugated beings who we can freely dominate however we like, consequently leading to us exterminating en masse dozens of genera and species in our pre-agricultural days and then creating a farming system that has caused such extreme suffering and death. So, as we look to our future, we must look to our past – not because we should return to it but to show us why we must move forward in a new direction entirely. One that doesn't just involve a different system of agriculture but that also involves reshaping our relationship with animals in general and no longer viewing them as simply existing for us to dominate as we please.

3.

THERE'S NO SUCH THING AS A HAPPY FARM ANIMAL

Outside of a slaughterhouse on a cold winter's morning, a farmer pulled up to the entrance. He was towing a trailer, inside which were several pigs. As he waited for the workers to let him in, I stood and spoke to him through his wound-down car window. He assured me that he absolutely cared about the pigs and that their wellbeing had always been the most important thing to him. I asked him if their imminent slaughter was the best thing for their wellbeing and constituted care. He looked at me, told me to step back from the side of the car and proceeded to drive in. I peered through a gap in the gates and watched as a worker, whose white overalls displayed a long smear of blood across the front, proceeded to force the pigs out of the trailer and through an open door and into a building that represents the antithesis of love. A place where not even hope can be found.

It is really appealing to believe the narrative that animal products come from happy animals who live a great life and are treated with care and respect. It eases our conscience as consumers and reinforces the idea that buying animal products is not a moral concern. We want to believe that any farmers who are exposed for abusing their animals are simply bad apples and don't represent an inherent, systemic problem.

The reality is there is no such thing as happy exploitation, happy mutilations or happy forced impregnations. And there is no such thing as a happy farm animal, as abuse and exploitation is an inherent and fundamental part of what we do to animals, regardless of how they are farmed. It is easy to allow ourselves to think that the labels and assurances that we give to animal products must mean something significant, but the notion of animal welfare can never really hold an animal's best interests at heart, as its purpose is to facilitate the continuation of animal exploitation in a way that remains profitable. These labels may make us feel better as consumers, but every animal will still one day meet the knife hanging in the slaughterhouse.

As a vegan who was brought up in England, I am often reminded that the UK has among the highest animal welfare standards in the world and told that while it is understandable to be against the US system of intensive factory farming, British family-run farms abide by our high standards, so I needn't worry. Everyone knows bad things happen to animals in other parts of the world, is the implication, but we would never allow animal abuse in this country.

Ironically, in every country I have ever visited, I have always met people who have told me that their animals are treated better than they are anywhere else, including in the USA, where I was defiantly told that in Texas they have the best animal husbandry practices in the world. This exceptionalism is not, therefore, something that only exists in the UK. That said, there is some truth in the statement that the UK has some of the highest animal welfare standards. In global rankings, the UK, Switzerland, Austria, the Netherlands, Denmark and Sweden are the best in the world when it comes to animal welfare laws.[1]

Unfortunately, this makes what happens even more damning, because it is not the ranking that is important but what occurs in the countries at the top of those rankings. So, it is worth noting that everything that is mentioned in this chapter (unless otherwise stated) occurs in a country that is considered one of the best in the world – meaning that when it comes to the lives of farmed animals, this is as good as it gets. It is also worth saying that what follows in this chapter is far from comfortable and much of what is discussed is difficult to read and extremely upsetting, but it is important to understand the reality of what is happening and what we are paying for when we buy animal products. While it may be unpleasant for us to read about how badly animals are treated, it's far more unpleasant for them to have to experience it. The animals can't simply skip this chapter (which of course you can); this is what they are forced to endure.

DON'T TRUST THE RED TRACTOR

In the UK, there are a number of schemes intended to reassure consumers that the animal products they buy are sourced from reputable farms with high animal welfare standards. But do welfare schemes such as Red Tractor and RSPCA Assured actually safeguard the animals and ensure that they are treated well?

The Red Tractor label is the UK's largest animal welfare certification scheme and, in their own words, is supposed to assure us that the 'animals have been well cared for'. It is a huge selling point for farmers and a source of reassurance for consumers, with the sticker of approval proudly displayed on just about every animal product that comes from a British farm. However, what many people are not aware of is that the Red Tractor scheme was set up by the National Farmers'

Union (NFU) and it is owned by the NFU and other industry bodies such as Dairy UK. On their board, which is in charge of developing Red Tractor's standards, there are, among others, members who have worked for some of the largest meat companies in Europe, a board member who is also the CEO of the powerful lobby group the British Meat Processors Association and a member who is also the agricultural director for Avara Foods Limited, a joint venture between Faccenda Foods Limited and Cargill. These companies are the largest producers of chicken, turkey and duck products in the UK, and conditions on their farms are regularly exposed as being horrendous for the animals, with violations of Red Tractor standards routinely documented. Are we really expected to believe that an audit from an inspector is going to provide any real accountability for a farm that is owned by a company whose agricultural director also sits on the board of the organisation that is auditing it?

As Red Tractor was set up by the NFU, an organisation funded by the membership fees of farmers, the same farmers it is supposed to be auditing, it is, in essence, an assurance scheme run by the very people it is supposed to hold accountable. It was also set up following the BSE crisis in the 1990s specifically to reassure consumers at a time when trust in the UK agricultural system had been eroded, which, ironically, happened because of farming practices that were encouraged by the animal farming industries, the same industries that now run the Red Tractor scheme. It is nothing other than a smokescreen created by the very industry we, as consumers, believe it is holding accountable.

Red Tractor boast that they perform 60,000 audits on farms each year; however, an investigation revealed that as few as 0.08 per cent of those visits were unannounced.[2] In the case of Lambrook pig farm in Somerset, for example, which was the subject of a national press exposé that discovered dead and living pigs covered in excrement and pigs held in tiny concrete pens and tethered with chains hanging from the ceiling, Red Tractor had audited the farm and passed it as acceptable. This means that the farm had cleaned up its act for the inspection that was expected, or Red Tractor simply turned a blind eye to what they saw. Either situation provides a damning indictment of the legitimacy of the scheme itself.

The Red Tractor assurances only meet the basic requirements and do not go meaningfully beyond anything other than what is required by law, and yet their logo is plastered all over animal products as if it signifies something important. At its core, all the label means is that the product in question comes from a farm that isn't operating illegally. And sometimes not even that is true, as Red Tractor-approved farms have been exposed for illegally electrocuting animals,[3] for breaking the necks of animals and leaving them convulsing on the floor while still alive,[4] for deliberately stamping on and throwing animals,[5] and much more. In fact, illegal practices have been documented on farms that have passed multiple Red Tractor audits,[6] again making a complete mockery of the scheme and its auditing process.

Once you see the Red Tractor label for what it really is, the whole illusion of animal farming begins to slip. This is the reality of the facade that we have been presented with.

THE PARADOX OF THE RSPCA

Despite the protection of animals being their core purpose, the Royal Society for the Prevention of Cruelty to Animals (RSPCA), founded in 1824 and arguably the largest animal welfare organisation in the world, is not much better. In the early 1990s, the RSPCA created the Freedom Food welfare scheme, which was meant to ensure that farmed animals were given five freedoms: from hunger and thirst; from discomfort; from pain, injury or disease; from fear and distress; and to express normal behaviour. The scheme, however, regularly drew criticism, as the requirements for farmers to be RSPCA certified did not guarantee the list of objectives were met and still allowed – as examples among many others – mutilations such as tail docking, teeth clipping and castration, and the rearing of animals intensively indoors. The Farm Animal Welfare Committee (FAWC), an independent advisory body set up by the UK government, later stated that the five freedoms were merely 'ideal states' or aspirations, as opposed to 'standards for acceptable welfare',[7] which is a position that the RSPCA has reiterated in their guidelines as well.

In 2015, the RSPCA rebranded their Freedom Food label, changing it to RSPCA Assured, removing the five freedoms and instead opting to approve farms if they meet their farm animal welfare standards. The RSPCA doesn't state how many of their farm audits are unannounced. Instead, they state that 'to make sure that someone is on-site when the assessor arrives, we book the assessment in advance'.[8] They also perform 'informal check-ins'. These aren't assessments but instead consist of the RSCPA's farm livestock officers providing advice on different farming practices and how best to implement the standards. The RSCPA only has five of these officers covering the entire UK.[9] Furthermore, farmers have to pay an annual membership to become part of the welfare scheme, meaning that the RSPCA is auditing farmers who financially support them.

The RSPCA have certified around 70 per cent of Scottish salmon farms but also revealed in 2020 that they were paid more than £500,000 by Scottish salmon farmers.[10] Not to mention that the RSPCA's farmed salmon advisory groups, which exist to provide advice on fish welfare, are filled with people from the fish farming industries. This means that the RSPCA's welfare guidance for fish farming is being very heavily influenced by the fish farming industries themselves. This becomes even more concerning when viewed alongside an investigation into 22 Scottish salmon farms that was carried out by Compassion in World Farming and released in 2021. The investigation documented farms owned by producers who also sit on the RSPCA's advisory groups and revealed severe levels of sea-lice infestations, open wounds and high numbers of on-farm mortalities, with bins and open pits filled with dead salmon.[11] Many of the farms had also been given RSPCA Assured certification previous to the investigation and following the investigation retained their certification.

Astonishingly, the RSPCA have even certified salmon farms where employees were shooting seals to stop them from eating the fish they were farming, with the RSPCA's head of campaigns stating in 2018 that 'seal shooting is not culling, it's about pest control'.[12] Thankfully, the practice of shooting seals was outlawed in the UK in early 2021. However, this came about not because salmon farmers wanted to stop killing seals, or because the RSPCA was campaigning to end the practice, or even because the Scottish government (who handed out licences to allow it to happen) realised that it was wrong. It was made illegal because there were fears that the USA, which accounts for 26 per cent of Scotland's salmon exports, would ban the import of Scottish salmon as shooting seals would break their wild marine mammal welfare laws.[13]

It's not just the RSPCA's technical advisory groups for the salmon industry that are of concern. Their chicken standards technical advisory group has members who also hold senior positions at Moy Park and 2 Sisters Food Group, two of the largest chicken companies in the UK, and their laying hen standards technical advisory group includes members from the egg industry, including the chairman of the British Egg Industry Council (BEIC), who is also the technical director of Noble Foods – the largest egg producer in the UK. The BEIC was set up to represent the egg industry, and its members are the 11 major egg companies in the UK. So, the chairman of a council that exists to best serve the egg industry is also a member of the laying hen advisory group for the UK's leading animal welfare charity.

The actions of the RSPCA have allowed cruel practices to be inflicted on animals while simultaneously alleviating the concerns of consumers about those practices. The RSPCA is meant to be for animals what the National Society for the Prevention of Cruelty to Children (NSPCC) is for children. But while the NSPCC works to end cruelty to children, the RSPCA works to normalise cruelty to animals and even profits from it by receiving funds to hand out certifications to those carrying out the acts of cruelty.

When discussing the guidelines for farmed animals, a representative from RSPCA Assured stated that standards have 'got to be commercially viable'.[14] In essence, the animals are involved in a non-consensual compromise where any consideration for their lives must be weighed against the financial burden such a consideration will incur on the farmers. This statement is effectively an admission that the RSPCA is fully aware that the guidelines they create aren't what's actually best for the animals.

The RSPCA has stated that they believe that it is better for them to work within the industry,[15] but it seems highly unlikely that there will be RSPCA Assured Labrador steaks or RSPCA Assured minced poodle anytime soon. In fact, the RSCPA has been working in China to end the dog meat trade, not to make it RSPCA Assured.[16] Plus, that argument is obviously deeply flawed when viewed alongside the idea of the NSPCC working with child abusers or anti-human traf-ficking charities working with traffickers. The farming of animals may be legal while the abuse of children and human trafficking clearly isn't, but that's really beside the point – a charity seeking to prevent cruelty should be doing exactly that.

However, the RSPCA finds itself stuck between a rock and a hard place. It is a charity reliant on public donations and philanthropic offerings, and if it began to campaign against the consumption of animal products, it would risk alienating most of its financial supporters. However, this means that its work is less concerned with ending cruelty to animals and more about courting public opinion. So the question remains: is the RSPCA genuinely interested in preventing cruelty to animals, or is it simply creating policies around social norms, even though those norms are in fact perpetuating cruelty to animals?

Unfortunately, the RSPCA does very little when breaches of welfare are committed and animal agriculture workers are found to be breaking the law. In the case of Hoads Farm, an egg farm in Sussex, the RSPCA initially removed their certi-fication following footage that revealed ill and deformed birds and dead hens in varying stages of decomposition left around the farm. They then reinstated the certification even though the farm had not only broken the RSPCA guidelines but had also broken the law, as it is supposed to be illegal to neglect a farm animal.[17] The farm was reinstated with special measures (they would receive unannounced visits), but at the very least it should have had to show compliance with the rules and guidelines before regaining its certification. Instead, they received no punishment and didn't even lose their certification.

This is all part of a systemic problem with animal farming oversight. Even when farms break the law, they are hardly ever punished by the legal system for doing so. While the RSPCA is meant to be creating accountability, it is often financially incentivised to not prosecute farmers. This is because the charity's reputation would be brought into question if it did, as it would reveal the failings in its oversight and animal welfare management. Instead, the RSPCA can simply say that the farms have been visited and the organisation is now satisfied that they are compliant, meaning nobody is prosecuted and the RSPCA goes on receiving fees from farmers for keeping them certified and at the same time further reassuring the public that there is nothing to be concerned about.

ANIMAL CRUELTY IS NOT A CASE OF ONE BAD APPLE

Unfortunately, situations of law breaking and welfare breaches are anything but uncommon. According to an investigation by the Bureau of Investigative Journalism, there were more than 9,500 recorded animal welfare breaches in the UK between July 2014 and June 2016 at slaughterhouses alone, including nearly 4,500 category four breaches, which are the most serious.[18] However, meat inspectors stated that this number was not truly representative, as inspectors are often intimidated into not reporting breaches or simply don't witness them. These breaches included chickens being boiled alive, pigs being submerged alive in tanks of scalding-hot water, animals not being stunned properly or even at all before slaughter, and trucks of animals suffocating or freezing to death. A single breach can involve hundreds of animals, as was the case when nearly 600 chickens died after being left in very hot conditions in the truck in which they had been taken to the slaughterhouse.

The investigation by the Bureau of Investigative Journalism stated that, 'Many animals are presented for slaughter in appalling condition – the records show some emaciated or too weak to stand, others diseased or suffering from fractures and open wounds. Failures in stunning procedures – which can result in animals regaining consciousness before being killed – are commonplace.' Regardless of this, a lawyer working on behalf of the meat industry complained that the rules requiring a permanent veterinarian presence in slaughterhouses were too 'stringent'.[19]

A group called Animal Aid investigated 15 slaughterhouses in England and published their findings in a report in 2017.[20] They filmed the law being broken in 14 of these slaughterhouses, including workers punching animals, burning them with cigarettes and deliberately electrocuting them. In two slaughterhouses, nearly every single pig was improperly stunned. The one slaughterhouse that didn't break the law during the three days of filming that took place there was still deemed by the Foods Standards Agency (FSA), the organisation that oversees slaughterhouses, to have been implementing poor practices.

The reality is, we've been told so often that we treat animals humanely that we assume malpractice or illegal abuse must be a rarity and that the standard legal practices can't be that bad. But unfortunately, abuse of animals is simply systemic and legally condoned, and, from the perspective of the animals, the legal practices also cause them suffering, pain and fear. So how do we farm animals and what exactly do these standard practices look like?

THE REALITY BEHIND A BACON SANDWICH

It is estimated that around 1.5 billon pigs are killed globally each year, with the vast majority being slaughtered in China and the USA.[21] The mother pigs, called sows, are impregnated either by being placed in a pen with a boar or through artificial insemination, where semen is usually obtained by a boar mounting a dummy and a worker acquiring the semen by hand. A device, called a 'breeding buddy', is then placed on the back of the sows to stimulate them before a worker places a catheter inside their cervixes and begins the process of inserting the semen.

In the UK, the use of gestation crates was banned in 1999; however, in countries such as the USA, Canada and China, they are still used as standard practice. The EU also only has a partial ban on their use, meaning sows can still be kept in the crates for up to ten weeks every year. A gestation crate is a tiny metal cage that measures roughly the same length and width of the pregnant pigs, meaning that once in the crate the sows are unable to turn around and are restricted to being able to stand up and lie down. The pigs will spend their entire pregnancy, which is around 16 weeks, inside these crates. Underneath the sows is concrete flooring, with the back section slatted, which they defecate and urinate through. In the stalls, the sows display signs of extreme stress and frustration – unsurprisingly, as these highly intelligent animals for weeks on end can only spend their time endlessly biting on the bars, either to relieve their boredom or in the hope that they will one day break free. But they never do and they never will.

At the end of the sows' gestation periods, they are moved to farrowing crates, which are essentially the same as gestation crates, with the pigs being unable to turn around, with the addition of a section to the side of the cage to allow the piglets to suckle from their mothers. The mother pigs will live in the farrowing crates for up to five weeks. Their piglets are separated from them around four weeks after they have been born. In the UK, farrowing crates are still legal and are considered standard practice. The National Pig Association (NPA) has even been working to ensure that a ban on farrowing crates isn't implemented in the UK, with the chairman of the NPA stating in 2021 that they had been attempting to 'steer government towards sensible practical solutions' in order to 'avoid a repeat' of the banning of gestation crates in the late 1990s.[22]

Farmers say that farrowing crates are used to stop the sows from crushing their piglets; however, research has shown that there is no difference in piglet mortality between those whose mothers are kept in the crates and those who are not.[23] In reality, farrowing crates allow farmers to house more pigs in less space and are more cost efficient, a point the chairman of the NPA implied himself when discussing his opposition to a potential ban on the crates, stating that he feared producers would be forced to exit the industry if more costly alternatives had to be found.[24]

After the piglets have been weaned, the sows are usually impregnated again within a couple of weeks and the process repeats. This cycle of impregnation and incarceration continues for around three to five years, at which point the sows are taken to the slaughterhouse to be killed for cheap pork products, like pies and pastries. I used to love sausage rolls and would get them all the time, never once considering that they are made from the ground-up body parts of multiple mother pigs.

Piglets usually have their teeth clipped out and their tails chopped off without the use of any anaesthetic as soon as they are born. The mutilations are carried out to reduce incidences of pigs attacking one another or cannibalising, both of which are consistent problems in pig farms due to the confinement of the pigs and the subsequent frustration and boredom they endure. The fact that the farmers mutilate the piglets to prevent these behaviours is in essence an acknowledgement that they know the farming causes the pigs psychological and physical distress. Routine tail docking of pigs is actually illegal, but an estimated 81 per cent of piglets in the UK are still docked anyway.[25] Castration is not banned in the UK but is uncommon. However, it is still standard practice in most countries around the world, with newborn piglets being castrated with a scalpel. This is done to avoid something called boar taint, which creates an unpleasant taste and smell in the meat. To get around this problem, pigs in the UK are slaughtered at a younger age.

When the piglets are separated from their mothers, they are moved to fattening pens, which are normally concrete or metal pens with slats in the floor for the pigs to defecate and urinate through. Even outdoor-reared pigs spend half their lives being farmed inside, often in slatted pens; the only difference is that for the first half of their lives they have access to the outside. This doesn't mean they have access to pasture, though, as pens can still be concreted as long as they are not fully enclosed inside and provide access to an outside area and some fresh air. Outdoor bred means the piglets are born outside but are then brought inside after they are weaned (at around four weeks) to be fattened. It is estimated that only 3 per cent of pigs will spend their entire lives with access to outdoor space.[26] In outdoor-reared and outdoor-bred systems of pig farming, the sows are not kept in farrowing crates but are kept in huts with access to an outside area. A former Red Tractor CEO said in regards to outdoor-bred pork, 'The advantages are some people are prepared to pay more money for it because they think it's better welfare.'[27]

On the outdoor-reared and outdoor-bred farms I have visited, this translated to the sow being kept in a metal-gated area, which has a covered hut and some straw. They can turn around and walk about a little but the fact that they are kept in a marginally better situation than the sows housed in farrowing crates is hardly a consolation. While one system may be preferable to the other, neither are preferable objectively speaking – such is the paradox of animal welfare legislation. We are sold the idea that animal welfare is important because it means that we are not causing as much suffering to an animal as we could – but just because we can do something worse doesn't mean that what we are doing is OK. It's akin to making the claim that human exploitation in the garment industry is moral because the workers are given a cushion to sit on and a bottle of water.

It is also not unusual for pigs who are sick to be killed on farms. For adult pigs, the most common forms of on-farm death are being shot, either with a rifle or shotgun, or with the use of a captive bolt stunner.[28] The issue with the captive bolt is that legally it is only meant as a method of stunning and is not commonly used in slaughterhouses for pigs, as their suitable 'target areas' are very small and their brains lie deep in their heads, meaning that the bolts will often be ineffective at rendering them unconscious. This can result in multiple shots being required, causing intense suffering and trauma. However, because it is primarily designed to stun the animals, the pigs still often have to be killed as well. This can be done through a process called pithing, which is where a rod is thrust through the bolt hole in the skull and through the brain, down towards the tail, before being slid back and forth to cause damage to the brain and upper spinal cord. Alternatively, the pigs will be bled out, which is where they have their throats cut. Due to the ineffectiveness of the captive bolt, the animals can remain conscious throughout either process.

Piglets are often killed because they are too weak or are not growing fast enough. The most common form of 'humane' death for piglets on farms is a process referred to as external trauma, often informally known as 'thumping'. This involves the piglets receiving a sharp blow to the top of their heads, sufficient to break their skulls. The most common way that this is done is by the farmer lifting a piglet by their back legs and slamming their head down, either on the floor or against the wall. This process often needs to be repeated several times to ensure the piglet is dead, otherwise they can be left conscious but with severe haemorrhaging. An investigation on a UK farm revealed that workers were 'thumping' piglets against the bars of the crates housing their mothers,[29] and at a different UK farm workers were filmed using hammers.[30] This practice is not only legal but is defended by the National Pig Association, who refer to it as 'an effective and appropriate way of humanely killing a piglet'.[31] It is allowed by Red Tractor and the RSPCA as well.

Pigs are generally sent to a slaughterhouse to be killed at around five to six months old. They are transported in large haulier trucks, which can carry hundreds of pigs at a time. The animals can be kept in these trucks for up to 28 hours in the USA and Canada. During this time, they are denied access to food or water, and they are often transported during extreme weather conditions, with animals dying from heatstroke and heart attacks because of the intense heat or alternatively freezing to death during the winter.

Once at the slaughterhouse, there are two main methods of pig slaughter. The first is electrical stunning followed by exsanguination, which is where the pigs are hoisted by one of their back legs and have their throats severed. The electrical stunning is carried out by a current being applied to the head of the pig; unfortunately, because the animals are scared and will try to escape, it can be very difficult for slaughterhouse workers to apply the electric current in a way that causes unconsciousness. This can mean that the pigs either have to be stunned repeatedly, each time enduring a painful electric shock, or they are still conscious when they are then hoisted by their legs to have their throats cut, bleeding out while still awake.

After they have had their throats cut, the pigs are then transported down the kill line to the scalding tank, where they are lowered into very hot water that loosens their bristles and skin. It is not uncommon for pigs to still be alive when they enter the scalding tank, meaning that they drown in extremely hot water.

The other method of pig slaughter, which is regarded as the most humane in places like the UK, Australia and most of the European Union, is the use of a CO_2 gas chamber. Two or three pigs are loaded into a metal gondola that is lowered into a pit filled with carbon dioxide. The concentration of CO_2 is normally 80 per cent or higher, which is recognised as being highly toxic for pigs. In fact, it has been shown that concentrations above 20 per cent create a toxic reaction.[32] The carbon dioxide replaces the oxygen in the pigs, causing them to hyperventilate and thrash about in a state of panic as they lose consciousness. The CO_2 also forms an acid when it comes into contact with wet surfaces, such as the eyes, lungs and throats of the pigs, causing them pain and distress alongside the suffocation.[33] This process can take longer than 60 seconds. Disturbingly, in 2003, the UK government's animal welfare advisory body recommended that this practice should banned, but it has instead become more prevalent.[34] This is how 86 per cent of the pigs in the UK are slaughtered.[35]

Alternative gasses such as argon or nitrogen will also cause the pigs to lose consciousness and have been shown to cause less suffering. However, the process takes longer, meaning that the extra time as well as the higher cost of the gases make the alternatives unfeasible in the eyes of the pig meat industry.

It is worth stating, however, that the problem with pig slaughter is not solely the manner in which they are killed but the fact that they are killed at all. Even using a gas that would be less toxic wouldn't make the process moral or objectively humane. I have described the methods used to kill the pigs to illustrate how little regard these industries have for the animals and how disingenuously words such as 'humane' are used. At the end of the day, we have to ask ourselves how can the taste of bacon justify the exploitation, abuse and ultimately needless death the animals are forced to endure?

GOT CRUELTY? WHAT GOES INTO A GLASS OF MILK

Cows are mammals, which means that, like humans, they only produce milk once they've had a baby. So, from around 15 months old, cows begin the process of being impregnated, most commonly through artificial insemination. This is done by a farmer acquiring semen from a bull, normally by using a dummy cow and an artificial vagina that the farmer will manually guide the bull's penis into or through a process called electro-ejaculation, which involves the insertion of a device into the bull's rectum that delivers an electric shock. The farmer will restrain the cow in a device known as a cattle crush and then insert their arm inside her anus to hold her cervix in place through the lining of the anus before injecting the semen into her.

A cow's gestation period is around nine months. The newborn calf will take his or her first drink from their mother, as the first feed contains colostrum, which is full of nutrients and antibodies. However, once the newborn calf has drunk the colostrum, the farmer separates them from their mother, normally within the first 24 hours. This is done so that the farmer can take as much milk as possible to be sold for human consumption.

I have visited many dairy farms, both in the UK and abroad, but one experience in particular sticks out for me. I and several others had gone to a dairy farm with the permission of the farmers. As we were wandering around, we came across a pen, inside of which was a mother cow and her newborn baby. The baby was so newborn that the mother was still licking her clean. As we stood there, the farmer told us that he was about to separate them from each other. He then proceeded to bring in what was essentially a cage on wheels. He opened the door of the cage, picked up the calf and put them inside before closing the door and wheeling them off.

As soon as he walked away, the mother cow followed behind to see where he was taking her baby. I ended up walking with the mother as far as we were allowed to go. The farmer, still wheeling the mother cow's baby, walked through an open gate, stopped and then closed it on us both. The mother cow watched her baby being taken further and further away from her. She turned her head and looked at me, hoping I would open the gate so she could catch up.

There is something profoundly moving about looking into the eyes of an animal. You recognise that behind those eyes is someone who is having an experience and through that recognition you can empathise with that experience. The same is true when they are suffering. The mother cow looked directly at me, but I was completely useless and unable to do anything to help. The normalisation and legalisation of her suffering meant that she had no way of being reunited with her baby. She would never be able to escape from what we humans were doing to her.

Cows form a strong maternal bond with their children, and their herds are matriarchal. Consequently, the separation of the child from their mother causes them both deep psychological distress and grief. The mother cow will then be milked by the farmer two or three times a day, taking the milk that is meant to feed her child, before she is then forcibly impregnated again as the process repeats.

Dairy cows have been selectively bred, meaning that they produce up to ten times more milk than they naturally would. This places a huge amount of strain on their bodies, increasing their risk of developing mastitis and lameness. Due to the strain placed on their bodies through the milking and calving processes, mother cows will sometimes do the splits, where their back legs splay out. In the event of this happening, a farmer will use a chain, called a hobble, to shackle their back legs together.

When we think of dairy cows, we think of cows grazing in fields, and that is true for many of them in the UK, albeit only for a certain part of the year due to weather limitations. However, around 20 per cent of UK dairy cows are farmed in zero-grazing systems,[36] and in the USA the majority are kept in such facilities, with the USDA estimating that 40 per cent of US dairy cows are housed in tie stall systems,[37] which is where they are restrained in individual stalls. In Canada, that figure is 75 per cent,[38] and more than a third of dairy cows in Germany are housed in tie stalls.[39]

Due to the strain placed on their bodies, cows become infertile and too weak or too ill after around five to seven years, significantly less than their natural twenty-year lifespan. When they are no longer profitable for the farmer, the cows are deemed to be a financial burden and not worthy of life and are taken to the slaughterhouse. The most common method of slaughter is a cow being forced into a stun box, where the slaughterhouse worker will then use a captive bolt gun to render her unconscious. Due to the precision required, and the fact that the cows will move around and try to escape, it is very common for the captive bolt to be used ineffectively. This results in either multiple bolts to their head being applied or the cow still being conscious as she is then released from the stun box to be shackled by one of her back legs. Once shackled, the cow will have her throat cut, which will then cause her to bleed to death before she is transported down the kill line to begin the process of being skinned and butchered. Disturbingly, there are many accounts from workers describing cows arriving at the butchering stage while still alive, meaning their bodies have been cut open and their skin peeled off before they have died.

About half of all the beef consumed comes from the dairy industry.[40] So while I did not realise it at the time, replacing meat with halloumi when I went vegetarian wasn't stopping cows from being slaughtered. The truth is, the dairy industry is very much the meat industry, just with the added years of cruelty before the cows reach the slaughterhouse.

It is estimated that in Europe around 3 per cent of dairy cows sent to slaughter are in the last trimesters of their pregnancies, meaning that they have babies inside of them that could be capable of independent life.[41] Because of this, the RSPCA has a set of guidelines on what should happen in the event of a pregnant cow being brought to slaughter. They state that the cow should be killed in the normal way but should then be left hanging on the kill line for at least five minutes to allow the foetus to die. However, sometimes the slaughterers don't know the cow is pregnant or they don't have time to wait – the kill line is constantly moving – or they wait the five minutes but the baby inside hasn't died. In these situations, the baby can fall out alive, conscious and gasping for air as their mother is being butchered.

In the event of this happening, the RSPCA states the baby should be killed 'with an appropriate captive bolt or by a blow to the head with a suitable blunt instrument'.[42] Their first and last experience of life is on the kill floor of a slaughterhouse, their mother hanging over them being butchered and cut apart as a worker approaches them to beat them to death with a blunt instrument. There is something profoundly wrong when the leading charity that is meant to protect animals is giving out instructions on how to kill an animal who has just been cut out of their dead mother. And remember, the UK is the best in the world when it comes to animal welfare.

Back on the farm, calves are separated from their mothers and placed in solitary confinement hutches. A so-called 'deluxe hutch' measures around 2 metres long, 1.2 metres wide and 1.4 metres high. The calves are legally allowed to be kept in these hutches for the first eight weeks of their life, although calves have been documented still living in these hutches at six months old, barely able to move and with sores on their backs from rubbing against the top of the crates.[43] They will also be mutilated by being disbudded, a process where their horn buds are burned out with a hot iron or eroded with a chemical.

After eight weeks, the calves will then be moved into group housing, where the females will begin the process of being incorporated into the herd to follow in the footsteps of their mothers, where they too will begin the cycle of being forcibly impregnated, having their babies separated from them and ultimately being killed in a slaughterhouse.

For the male calves, there are several options that a farmer can choose. First, they can raise them for veal. Many people are not aware that the veal industry only exists because of the dairy industry. In the EU, 6 million dairy calves are killed for veal each year, with the most common kind being so-called 'white veal'. This is created by the calves first being separated from their mothers and placed in solitary confinement hutches. They are then fed a low-iron diet, which can cause anaemia and is designed to keep their flesh pale. After the first two weeks of their lives, the farmers are not legally obliged to provide bedding, and the calves are typically housed on slatted floors, which makes lying down extremely uncomfortable.[44]

The calves are then raised in groups from eight weeks of age. They will spend the rest of their lives in these pens before they are taken to the slaughterhouse at around 20 to 24 weeks old. Like their mothers, the most common method of slaughtering calves is the use of a captive bolt gun before they are shackled by their legs and their throats are cut. The process is the same for 'rose veal', just without the low-iron diet and likely anaemia, and the calves are slaughtered when they are between 8 and 12 months old.

In the USA, it is estimated that around 450,000 to 700,000 calves are killed for veal each year with the majority of states still allowing the use of veal crates – tiny wooden boxes in which the calves are often unable to turn around and can even be chained by their necks to further reduce their movement. Just like in the EU, they are fed a low-iron diet, which, combined with the lack of mobility, is designed to keep their flesh supple. They can be raised in these crates for their entire life, which is around 18 weeks, at which point they will be sent to a slaughterhouse to be killed. Many are unable to even walk to their slaughter as their muscles are so severely underdeveloped.

In the UK, the demand for veal is much lower than it is in continental Europe, so many British dairy calves are transported through the live export system into Europe, where they will then be raised for veal. It is more common for dairy calves to be sold into the beef industry in the UK. However, dairy calves are a different breed to those raised specifically for beef, meaning they aren't as muscular or as financially desirable. Because of this, they are seen as 'low quality' and are therefore much more likely to be sold at livestock markets and raised in semi-intensive beef farms, which are typically farms where the cattle are raised solely inside. They will also be castrated, which is normally done by the farmer applying a tight rubber ring around the scrotum of the calf, restricting the blood flow and causing the testicles to fall off after a couple of weeks. The other most common method of castration is where the spermatic cords are crushed using a clamp called a burdizzo. However, shockingly, it is often not seen as economically viable for dairy calves to be sold to beef farms, as it can actually cost the farmer more money than just killing them. Consequently, around 60,000 to 95,000 male dairy calves are shot and discarded soon after being born in the UK every single year.[45]

Due to the negative public perception around this practice, supermarkets, dairy companies and Red Tractor are attempting to discourage it from happening. But the male calf problem doesn't suddenly go away simply because farmers are no longer allowed to shoot them. As a result, more farmers are now selling their calves to dealers who then take them to intensive beef farms or to slaughterhouses. An investigation in 2021 showed that calves as young as nine days old were left overnight on their own during winter in a slaughterhouse.[46] The next morning, at ten days old, they had their throats cut and were bled out. Their bodies were then incinerated or turned into products such as pet food or tallow, a substance that is used in the production of money, among other things. A ten-day-old baby, whose only experience of life is being taken away from their mother, loaded into a truck and driven to a slaughterhouse, is left in the cold overnight on a concrete floor before their throat is cut, all so we can pour their mother's milk over our cornflakes. If the colour of milk reflected the reality of the industry, it would run red with the blood of all the animals exploited and killed for dairy products.

WHERE'S THE BEEF? THE TRUE COST OF A BEEF BURGER

The first stage of beef production is calf rearing, where the cows being used for breeding are either artificially impregnated or are placed with a bull to get them pregnant. When the calves are born nine months later, they have their ears tagged and their horn buds removed using a hot iron or an erosive chemical. The males are castrated as well. In countries such as the USA, Canada and Australia, beef cattle are also often branded with a red-hot iron.

The process of cattle farming frequently involves the cattle being sold at auction markets and then transported to different farms. Auction markets are stressful environments where animals are kept in crowded pens as they wait to be sold. In the auction rooms that I have visited, the animals acted frantically, trying to find a way out. Instead, they are forced to stay in the pens by workers with paddles who guard the entrances and exits of the auctioning pens while the farmers bid on their bodies. I remember watching as the farmers observed the animals, not looking upon them as individuals but as objects, bidding for ownership of their lives based on aspects of their bodies such as their weight or build. It disturbed me that a room full of people could witness the clear signs of distress in front of them, but instead of working to stop it, they were actively perpetuating the system that caused it. The distress is so normalised that it's not even noticed.

After they have been weaned from their mothers, which is normally at around six to eight months old, calves are then typically taken elsewhere for the growing phase before then going into the 'finishing' phase, which can be on a different farm again. The purpose of this stage is to get the cattle to gain as much weight as possible in a short space of time, meaning that even in outdoor grazing systems the cattle will often be given some supplementary food to get them to slaughter weight. Interestingly, in the dairy industry, farmers will say that the reason they separate newborn calves from their mothers is because it is actually in the best interests of the mother and calf. Yet in the beef industry, where there is no financial incentive to separate the two, they are commonly allowed to remain together.

In countries such as the USA, Australia and Canada, feedlots are a common way of getting cattle to slaughter weight. Even animals who are raised in pastures are often 'finished' on grain in grassless pens where they are housed in large numbers, with some feedlots confining 85,000 cattle within them. They are deemed to be a more efficient and cost-effective way of getting cows to slaughter faster, as they require less land, and a grain diet allows the cattle to gain weight quicker.

In the UK, the number of US-style feedlots is on the rise, with herds of up to 3,000 cattle now being fattened by this method. Often the cattle will have spent time on pasture before being moved to the feedlots for the last quarter of their lives.[47]

Beef cattle are commonly slaughtered when they are between 12 and 24 months old but there have been calls from the National Beef Association for calves who are slaughtered at eight months old to be able to be labelled beef rather than veal. This is so that they can kill the animals earlier and not have to worry about consumers being less inclined to buy the product.[48]

Beef cattle are killed by being forced into a stun box and having a captive bolt shot into their head. A study into the stunning of cattle in the EU revealed that 12 per cent of cattle are shot more than once, and 14 per cent of calves were shot inaccurately.[49] In total, 12.5 per cent of cattle were deemed to have been inadequately stunned, meaning they will have been either fully or partially conscious as they had their throats cut. The study also showed that, on average, cattle don't have their throats cut until 105 seconds after being stunned, even though it is meant to happen within 60 seconds to ensure the animals don't regain consciousness.[50] As one ex-slaughterhouse worker in the USA put it when describing his experiences of seeing conscious animals on the kill line: 'I've seen thousands and thousands of cows go through the slaughter process alive. The cows can get seven minutes down the line and still be alive. I've been in the side-puller [a machine that peels the cattle's hides off] where they're still alive. All the hide is stripped out down the neck there.'[51] At another slaughterhouse, a USDA animal health technician even complained to his superiors: 'I complained to everyone – I said, "They're skinning live cows in there." Always it was the same answer: "We know it's true. But there's nothing we can do about it." '[52]

A few years before I became vegetarian, I started eating rare steak, and I would make comments about it being extra bloody, as if it was something to be proud of. But although I might have enjoyed eating steak with a steak knife, I would never have been the person to cut the animal's throat with a slaughterer's knife, and I certainly wouldn't have looked at my actions proudly if I saw just how bloody a piece of steak really is. While we might enjoy the taste of a burger or steak, such pleasure is trivial when stacked against the ethical cost of these products.

KENTUCKY FRIED CRUELTY: THE VIOLENCE IN A SHARING BUCKET

When I used to consume KFC, I never once stopped and thought consciously about the chickens I was eating. I'd order wings, but I never thought about the fact they were body parts or that for every two wings I ate one chicken had had to die. Or how a bucket contained multiple dead chickens, one meal equalling many lives. When we consider the sheer volume of chicken body parts we eat, it's perhaps not surprising that, apart from insects, they are the most abused and exploited terrestrial animal on the planet. Every year, around 66 billion are killed, which means that more than 180 million are killed every single day.[53]

Chickens have been selectively bred to reach slaughter weight by the time they are between 35 and 42 days old. This frequently leads to organ failure and leg problems as their bodies grow too fast for their joints and organs to keep up. Put into context, if a newborn human grew at the same rate as a farmed chicken, they would weigh 28 stone by their third birthday.[54] The life of a chicken raised for meat, referred to as a broiler chicken, is so horrible that the fact they are alive for such little time is a mercy. In the USA, more than 99.9 per cent of chickens are factory farmed,[55] while in the UK it is more than 95 per cent.[56]

Fertilised chicken eggs come from broiler breeding farms, where the males and females used for breeding are kept in indoor barns. Because the chickens grow so fast, farmers starve the birds so that they can slow the rate of growth and get as many fertilised eggs as possible from the hens. However, starving the birds causes them psychological distress and increases the incidence of abnormal behaviours such as aggression and feather pecking. The males are often mutilated as well by being debeaked, having the ends of their toes cut off and dubbed, which is where their combs are completely or partially removed. When the males and females are no longer suitable for breeding, they are slaughtered.

The fertilised eggs are then taken to hatcheries. The chicks hatch and are vaccinated before they are transported to the farms, where they are placed in barns that can hold as many as 50,000 birds.[57] In the UK, farmers will typically allow each bird an area less than the size of an A4 sheet of paper.[58]

I vividly remember the first time I ever visited a chicken farm. I was in the decontamination area that you had to go through before entering the main barn, and I looked through a window at what was inside. It was like watching something on TV – my brain couldn't comprehend what I was seeing. The barn seemed to be never-ending, extending far off into the distance, and the completely white floor was moving. It took me a second to realise that the entire floor was made up of tens of thousands of chickens who were so crammed together they had created what on first inspection looked more like a living carpet. I felt completely overwhelmed. If we see an animal suffering, we empathise with that one animal, but when we see thousands, it can be difficult to comprehend the experience each individual is having. But each animal in front of me was enduring their own individual experience of suffering. I then thought of all the other barns on the farm, each containing a similar number of individuals.

Legally, the barns are allowed to be windowless and artificially lit, which means the farmers can better control the environment. The farmers encourage the birds to eat more feed and grow larger by altering the lighting, with research showing that 20 hours of light a day creates the highest growth rate in the birds.[59] Every time I have visited a chicken farm, the lights have always been on, even when it's the middle of the night. However, Red Tractor standards in the UK mean that by 2023 a barn will need windows that equate to 3 per cent of its floor area.

On that first visit, I proceeded to open the door into the main section of the barn and tentatively took my first steps, the chickens in front of me flapping their wings and struggling to move as I cautiously stepped around them. These particular chickens were nearly ready to be 'harvested', an industry term meaning the birds were only a few days away from being sent to slaughter. The term 'harvested' is a good example of how desperately the industry tries to hide behind euphemisms.

As soon as I opened the door, I was hit by the thunderous noise of the ventilation system, which created an unrelenting wall of sound that was only matched by the loud chirping emitted by the tens of thousands of birds that surrounded me. As I continued to walk through the barn, I sank into the mounds of faeces that covered the entire floor, nearly causing me to lose my shoes and biosecurity shoe covers on several occasions. The barns are only cleaned when the chickens have been sent to slaughter, which means that every day the mounds of faeces pile up, and by the six-week mark every step you take is either onto a chicken or into excrement.

This build-up of faeces causes the air to become acrid with ammonia. The hazardous gas damages the respiratory systems and eyes of the birds, which can lead to lesions in their corneas partially or completely blinding them.[60] The ammonia can also cause something called hock burns, which are burns around their knee joints that come from them standing in faeces all day. The ammonia can also scorch off the feathers on their undersides, leading to painful red burns across their chests.

As I wandered around the barn, everywhere I looked there were chickens laid on their backs unable to move, pinned down by their own weight, gasping at the ammonia-filled air as their organs failed and they slowly died. Other chickens had their legs splayed due to their weight, rendering them unable to move. These animals would die from starvation and dehydration, unable to reach the water and feed points situated around the barn. There were also dead birds in different stages of decomposition, some who had died earlier that day and others who had died many days earlier. Some had rotted so much that they were featherless and semi-buried under faeces.

Farmers are supposed to work their way through each barn daily and pick out the dead birds and cull the ones who are close to death. They do this by either stamping on them, bludgeoning them or by swinging them around by their necks to break them. It's hard to know exactly how many chickens die on the farms, but the estimated on-farm mortality rate in the UK is 4 per cent,[61] which if the same was true worldwide would mean that for every 180 million chickens killed each day in slaughterhouses another 7.2 million chickens will have also died on farms. In many ways, the ones who die on farms are the lucky ones.

There is only suffering in chicken production, every second of every day. These animals are bred specifically to grow as fast as possible and then die. Even ones that are rescued and taken to an animal sanctuary will normally die within a matter of months. Their bodies are simply not meant to last. A chicken farmer who says they care about their chickens is akin to a tobacco company saying they care about people getting lung cancer.

For the birds who survive to slaughter age, teams of catchers then work their way through the barns, roughly picking up the chickens and forcing them into crates, which are then loaded onto trucks that take them to the slaughterhouse. It is estimated that in the UK alone, nearly one million chickens die on the way to the slaughterhouse each year, often because they are crushed in the crates and suffocate to death or because their bones have been broken and dislocated due to being handled roughly.[62]

Once in the slaughterhouse, the birds are killed in one of two ways. First, they can be loaded into gas chambers and suffocated using a mixture of gasses such as carbon dioxide and nitrogen. The progressive suffocation can lead to convulsions, gasping, vigorous wing flapping and panic.[63] Alternatively, they are shackled upside down by their feet onto a conveyor belt, which then carries them through an electrified water bath that is supposed to stun them before they then have their necks dragged over a rotating blade that cuts their throats. Due to the speed of the line, some birds do not make contact with the electrified water bath and can be conscious when they have their necks pulled over the blade. Other times, the blade might not cut their necks properly, meaning the animals are still alive when they are submerged into the scalding tank where their feathers are loosened.

Free-range chickens are often breeds that have a slower growth rate, meaning that they are kept alive for longer. But that normally only translates to them being alive for 56 days, which is just two to three weeks longer than conventionally raised broilers.[64] They also have daytime access to an outside area for at least half of their lives, but that only has to equal one square metre of space per bird, and a farmer can house roughly 13 free-range chickens per square metre of space indoors, which is compared to the roughly 17 birds per square metre of space that is permitted on a conventional Red Tractor farm. They are also killed in exactly the same way.

As I made my way out of the chicken farm, I looked into the barn one last time, the heat and the sound hitting me like a wave as pangs of guilt for all the individuals I had once forced to live their short, terrible lives in these barns came over me. I closed the door behind me, sealing the chickens back in their eternal prison. At that moment, I couldn't help but feel complicit in the system I sought to oppose. In the eyes of all the birds, I was the same as their abusers. After all, they were still there, although not for much longer. The catchers would soon be arriving.

WHY THERE'S NO SUCH THING AS A GOOD EGG

Hens raised for their eggs are a different breed than those raised for their meat, which means that they won't grow to be the same size. So male chicks are useless to the egg industry and are considered a by-product, their lives deemed to be worthless. Because of this, when the chicks are born in hatcheries, they are separated based on their sex. The males are put on one conveyor belt and the females are placed on another. The conveyor belt for the males then usually goes to one of two places: a gas chamber where they are gassed to death or an industrial macerator that grinds them up alive. This happens in all systems of egg farming, including free range and organic. In some countries, male chicks are alternatively suffocated in bin bags or crushed to death.

The other conveyor belt takes the female chicks to a machine that debeaks them. They are then loaded onto trucks that take them to growing sites, where they stay for about 16 weeks before being taken to the laying farms. In the UK, about 42 per cent of egg-laying hens are kept in cages,[65] and globally about 60 per cent are caged.[66] Caged hens are entitled to slightly more space than the size of a sheet of A4 paper each, meaning they are unable to stretch out their wings. They are also forced to stand on wire mesh, which they defecate through. If a hen gets picked on or becomes the victim of a more aggressive hen, they are unable to escape.

The other main system of egg farming is free range. When we see a box of free-range eggs, we may believe that these eggs must come from hens who lived a good life and didn't suffer. Before I was vegan, that's what I thought. I thought that you had a choice between buying caged and causing suffering or buying free-range and giving hens a nice life, so I always bought free range. I eventually realised that this is not the case. Free-range hens must have access to an outside space during the day; however, inside the barns, farmers are legally allowed to house nine birds per square metre of space.[67]

Because egg-laying hens have been selectively bred, they lay around 300 eggs a year, which places an extreme amount of stress on their bodies. Both caged and free-range hens can suffer from broken bones due to their calcium reserves being diverted to making the shells of their eggs. A survey of 67 flocks in the UK showed that the rates of fractures in non-cage systems was anywhere from 45 to 86 per cent.[68] Osteoporosis is also a problem, with it being estimated that 30 per cent of the total mortality of hens in cages is linked to the condition.[69]

The hens can suffer from respiratory disease and egg peritonitis, which is where a hen's reproductive system becomes inflamed and infected, often because an egg hasn't formed properly and has become infected with E. coli. Prolapses can also occur from the excessive amount of egg laying, and skin diseases such as red-mite infestations and ammonia burns are common.

In many countries, a process called forced moulting is allowed, which is essentially where the farmers put the hens on a starvation diet that makes them lose their feathers. This is done to force the hens to grow fresh feathers, which works to rejuvenate their reproductive systems, leading to larger eggs afterwards. It's a way in which farmers can maximise the amount of money that can be made from the hens' bodies before they eventually go to slaughter.

Once an egg-laying hen is about 72 weeks old, her egg production declines, meaning that the farmer no longer sees the benefit of keeping her alive. As a result, egg-laying hens are then loaded into crates, placed on trucks and taken to slaughterhouses, where they will be killed in the same way as the chickens who are raised just for their flesh. All egg-laying hens that don't die on farms are killed in slaughterhouses and turned into cheap meat products.

FORCING LAMBS TO THE SLAUGHTER

One of the first times I ever saw a lamb up close was outside a slaughterhouse in Somerset. They were lying dead on the floor outside the entrance to the kill floor. There was a pool of blood that had formed around the sheep's face, suggesting they had suffered a head injury. In the holding pen just next to the dead lamb were several dozen more lambs. These ones were alive, though, waiting for the worker to open the door and force them through it one by one.

When the worker entered, the lambs moved as far back from him as they could. He began pushing and shoving them through the door, causing them to jump over one another in a desperate attempt to delay the inevitable. After a dozen or so lambs had entered into the building, he followed them in and closed the door, leaving the remaining lambs outside waiting for the same process to happen again. A nearby conveyor belt, which began inside the building but carried objects out through a hole in the wall and dropped them into the courtyard, started moving.

After only a few minutes its purpose became clear. The skin of a lamb emerged through the wall, falling onto the ground. The next one appeared and then the next. After the last skin had emerged, a worker came to move them so they could later be turned into items like sheepskin rugs. The door to the holding pen then opened again and the worker began forcing the next dozen lambs into the building.

Lamb and sheep farming is often viewed as the most idyllic form of farming. However, just because we see sheep grazing in the fields doesn't mean that they don't suffer, and it doesn't change the fact they too have their lives needlessly taken from.

Artificial insemination of sheep is more complicated than with most other farmed animals, which means that many countries such as the UK mainly breed sheep using rams. However, in countries such as Australia and New Zealand, artificial insemination is widely practised in the sheep industry. This first requires semen to be obtained from a ram. Most commonly this is done by restraining a ewe and coaxing a ram to mount her; however, the farmer will then place the ram's penis into an artificial vagina instead. The other method is through electro-ejaculation.

The process of insemination then involves a ewe being clamped down onto a trolley, which positions her on her back with her underbelly exposed. The inseminator then makes two incisions, one on each side of her stomach, before inserting a scope into one side to see inside the ewe. Gas is often pumped inside her in order to displace the intestine, stomach and bladder so that the inseminator can better view the womb. He then takes the semen and injects it through the other incision and into the uterine horn of the ewe.

A ewe's gestation is around five months, at which point she will give birth to one or two lambs, although some breeds average more than two lambs per litter because of selective breeding. In the event that some of the lambs die, farmers will carry out a process called grafting, which is essentially

the act of getting a ewe to adopt a lamb that is not biologic-
ally hers. The preferred method of grafting is for the farmer
to skin the dead lamb and place their skin over a living,
orphaned one.

Male lambs are castrated, normally by a rubber ring that
is secured around the base of the scrotum until it falls off.
However, there are also other legally permitted methods,
such as surgical castration, which involves cutting the testes
out of the scrotum. Both males and females will have their
tails docked, with the rubber-band method being commonly
used for tail removal as well. Other methods include the use
of a tail iron, where a heated blade is used to sever and cau-
terise the tail, and the clamp-and-surgical-removal method,
where a clamp is used to crush the bone in the tail and kill the
nerves. The tail is then left for a few days before being
removed using hot irons.

In Australia, the world's leading producer of wool, providing a quarter of all wool globally and 80 per cent of all
merino wool, the process of mulesing is standard practice.
Mulesing is a process in which a sheep is restrained on their
back and then has the flaps of skin around their backside cut
off. It is an incredibly painful procedure that leaves the lambs
with open wounds that take weeks to heal. The justification
for both mulesing and tail docking is that it is done to prevent flystrike, a condition where flies lay eggs in the moisture,
urine and faeces that is retained by the wrinkled skin around
the backside of the sheep. There are alternative non-surgical
methods that can be used; however, they require more management, and due to flock sizes most farmers are unwilling to
implement these less invasive methods, as they are more
effort and cost more.

The reason why flystrike is such a prevalent issue in the
first place is because sheep have been selectively bred to produce excessive amounts of wool. The more wrinkled a sheep

is, the more folds there are and the higher the volume of wool that is produced. It is often believed that it is ethical to wear wool because sheep need to be sheared. However, this is only true because we have selectively bred them in such a way that they no longer naturally shed their wool for the warmer months like wild sheep do. In essence, we have changed them physically to maximise the amount of money we can make from them, and then we mutilate them to try to reduce the incidence of a condition that is a problem precisely because we have selectively bred them. Then, to top it all off, we claim that the reason we mutilate them and literally carve off chunks of their skin is because we care about their wellbeing.

About 15 per cent of lambs who are born die, with some of the major causes including cold exposure and infectious diseases.[70] While we view sheep farming more positively because it involves outside grazing, farmers are unable to properly care for all the animals in their flock and accept the financial losses of dead lambs as being preferable to the extra management and expense that would be required to bring down lamb mortality. Many farmers also want to cash in on the spring lamb market, so they induce pregnancy earlier in the year than would be normal for sheep. This means that the lambs are born in winter, and many are unable to survive the freezing temperatures.

Lambs raised for their flesh are generally slaughtered at around five to eight months old. Lambs will either be sold directly to a slaughterhouse or they will go through the stressful environment of an auction market. Once at the slaughterhouse, the most common method of slaughter is the use of electrodes on a device that looks like a pair of tongs. The device is placed on either side of the lamb's head and electrocutes them. Alternatively, the lambs will be stunned by a captive bolt. They are then hung upside down and have their throats severed.

Although some lambs will be sheared before slaughter, there is less value in their wool, which often means that the cost of shearing will outweigh the price the farmer can get for selling the wool and is not therefore considered to be financially viable. Also, the meat can fetch a lower price if the lambs are bruised, which commonly happens during the shearing process. However, the skins of lambs are used and sold, often as single pelts, referred to as sheepskin or lambskin, or turned into leather.

Sheep used for breeding and for their wool are kept alive for longer and will be sheared once or twice every year. The process of shearing is often touted as being a harmless process, sometimes even compared to a haircut. However, an investigation into more than 30 shearing sheds in the USA and Australia caught shearers punching, kicking and stomping on sheep, hitting them in the face with electric clippers and standing on their heads, necks and legs. It was a similar story in the UK, where an investigation into 25 shearing sheds showed animals being stamped on, kicked, slammed and choked. The process was so brutal that sheep were often cut open, which led to the shearers sewing them back up without any pain relief. These sheep will be kept alive until they are no longer deemed to be profitable enough, at which point they too will be sent to a slaughterhouse.

SCREAMING SILENTLY: THE TRUE HORROR OF FISH CONSUMPTION

Fish are the animals that we kill the most of by far. To put it into perspective, we kill approximately 80 billion land animals every year;[71] however, it is estimated that we kill somewhere in the region of 0.8 to 2.3 trillion wild fish and 51 to 167 billion farmed fish in the same period.[72]

We often view fish as being animals that have short memories, lack any form of notable intelligence and don't even have the capacity to feel pain; however, this is untrue. The nervous systems of fish are similar enough to those of birds and mammals to show that they do feel pain, and when fish experience something that would cause other animals physical pain, they behave in ways suggestive that they feel it. Fish will learn to avoid unpleasant experiences like electric shocks and painkillers reduce the symptoms of pain that they would otherwise exhibit. Even crustaceans such as prawns have demonstrated similar behaviours by responding to acid being brushed on their antennae, showing complex and prolonged movements that diminished when local anaesthetic was applied beforehand.[73] Studies such as these have led to a scientific panel for the European Union concluding that the evidence shows that fish do feel pain.[74] Moreover, fish have also been shown to have stress responses, with their cortisol levels becoming raised when they are taken out of water and placed in a bucket.

Fish have also been shown to act intelligently. They can be taught how to evade a trap and remember it a year later, and they can learn from each other, recognise other fish they've spent time with previously, know their place within fish social hierarchies and remember complex spatial maps of their surroundings. Fish also work together with different species of fish and show cooperation and trust, with fish remembering which other fish were cooperative or uncooperative.

In the commercial fishing industry, impaling live bait on hooks is common practice. Longline fishing uses hundreds or even thousands of hooks on a single line that might be anything from 50 to 100 kilometres long. On each of these hooks is often a fish who has been impaled through their face or body as a means to entice larger fish to eat them and get hooked themselves. Furthermore, when the larger fish take the bait, they are likely to remain caught for many hours before the line is hauled in.

Another method of catching wild fish involves gill nets, which are walls of fine netting in which fish become snared, often by the gills, which can lead to suffocation. If they don't die, they can remain trapped for many hours before the nets are pulled in. The other most common method is bottom trawling, where huge nets are dragged across the seafloor, trapping anything that gets in their way before then being hauled out of the water.

Fish caught in the wild are then dumped on fishing boats and will die either by suffocation, being crushed under the weight of all the other fish on top of them or through rupturing of their internal organs caused by the rapid pressure changes when they are hauled out of the water. The fish that are still living when they begin to be processed will die through a combination of suffocation and evisceration, when the animals are gutted alive.

Sometimes fish are put onto ice as they suffocate; however, this has been shown to increase the severity of their distress and causes them to suffer for longer, as even though the cold can paralyse them, scientific studies have shown that they remain conscious and can feel pain and stress. One study found that some fish can remain conscious for 20 to 40 minutes after they have been gutted, depending on how much of their body has been removed.[75] This is absolutely horrific. Fish suffer and feel pain and yet we butcher and gut them while they are still alive.

Aqua farming, which is the equivalent of factory farming for fish and is responsible for more than half of all fish consumed worldwide each year, involves fish spending their entire lives in underwater enclosures, normally either in sea cages or concrete tanks. Many species of fish that we consume are adapted to the open ocean and swimming long distances. Salmon in particular can travel thousands of miles but in fish farms they are confined in cramped areas where they can only swim around in circles for their entire lives. Farmed fish are bred by having their ovulation or release of sperm induced through hormone injections. They are then often killed and gutted for their eggs or, in the case of the males, killed and their semen squeezed out of them. Alternatively, fish farmers will take the live fish and force the eggs and semen out of them by squeezing along their abdomens.

Many species of farmed fish have also been selectively bred, including salmon, who have been altered to grow abnormally fast and consequently suffer from compromised immune systems, enlarged heads and breathing difficulties. Because of overcrowding in the cages, the fish are more susceptible to disease and suffer from stress and physical injuries such as fin damage, eye cataracts and spinal deformity, as well as parasitic infections. Due to the prevalence of parasites and disease, a device called a thermolicer, which pumps salmon through tubes and across metal rollers that are filled with water above 30 degrees Celsius, is used to remove the lice. However, research has shown that temperatures above 28 degrees cause behavioural responses in salmon indicative of pain.[76] The treatment has also been shown to cause gill damage, scale and skin loss, and brain haemorrhages. The thermolicer and another lice treatment called a hydrolicer, which is similar but instead uses water pressure to remove the lice, were, according to data from the Scottish government, responsible for killing more than 100,000 farmed Scottish salmon between August 2017 and January 2018 alone.[77]

However, death is not uncommon on fish farms, with as many as 20 million salmon dying prematurely in 2019 on

Scottish salmon farms alone.[78] Because of the high mortality rates, antibiotic use is rampant.

Fish are regularly handled roughly on aqua farms, and fish that are deemed too sick are taken out of the tanks and often bludgeoned to death. In a 2020 investigation of four rainbow trout farms in the UK, including one that supplies a company endorsed by Jamie Oliver, workers were filmed throwing live fish, kicking them and bludgeoning them with wooden batons.[79]

Crustacean farming also involves suffering, with female prawns enduring a mutilation called eyestalk ablation, where the farmer either cuts off the eyes of the female prawns or squeezes and pulls them off instead. Alternatively, farmers will tie threads around the base of the eyes so that the blood supply is cut off and they fall off after a few days. This is done to destroy the glands behind the eyes that control the maturing of the ovaries, which forces them to grow rapidly, meaning the females can be used for breeding faster.

Farmed fish are slaughtered by a range of methods, such as gassing with carbon dioxide or cutting their gills without stunning. Similar to wild-caught fish, some farmed fish are simply left to suffocate in air or on ice. Alternatively, some are killed by being electrically stunned or are hit over the heads before then being bled out. It is also worth mentioning that many farmed fish are carnivorous, including salmon and sea bass. This means that they can be fed wild-caught fish, and the production of farmed fish therefore also contributes to the suffering of wild fish as well.

The methods by which fish are both farmed and killed are arguably the least humane out of all the animals that we kill. Even though this is the case, they are often the animals whose suffering we most ignore. It is easy to turn a blind eye to what fish are forced to endure, but they are still forced to endure it nonetheless.

THE HUMAN COST

People often accuse vegans of valuing non-human animals over humans; after all, there are still human rights issues that we need to address and solve, so shouldn't we deal with those first before worrying about other animals? This argument of course overlooks the fact that animal rights and human rights aren't mutually exclusive, and we can instead work towards improving them both at the same time, but it also fails to address the cases of human exploitation within the animal exploitation industries. For example, human rights transgressions are rampant in the seafood industry, with tens of thousands of workers estimated to be victims of forced labour, human trafficking and debt bondage.[80] Seafood from this exploitation has been traced to retailers and restaurants in the USA, Europe and Asia.[81]

Residents living in areas around farms have been shown to have increased rates of respiratory health problems related to air pollution from gases such as ammonia.[82] A 2021 study revealed that 12,700 deaths occur a year in the USA because of pollution from animal farming.[83] While in India and Bangladesh, due to the chemicals required to turn cattle skin into leather, tannery workers suffer from health problems such as skin diseases, acid burns, corroded fingers, peeling skin, eye problems[84] and even sudden death,[85] with the chemicals also increasing their risk of cancer.[86]

But the problem of human exploitation within animal farming is an issue that exists everywhere and is as systemic as animal farming itself. Although we may not realise it, animal exploitation doesn't just make the world more violent for animals – it also makes the world more violent for us humans as well, further adding to issues of human suffering and exploitation.

It's common for people to question the ethics of someone who works in a slaughterhouse, and yet doing so overlooks the real reason why people work in these places: a lack of choice. Slaughterhouses are found in lower-income areas, where there are fewer job opportunities. It's one of the lowest-paid industrial jobs with one of the highest turnover rates. It is also an industry filled with worker exploitation.

An inquiry released in 2010 by the Equality and Human Rights Commission (EHRC) in the UK found practices that appeared to break the law in UK slaughterhouses, particularly on issues regarding health, safety and equality, with basic human rights being endangered. The commission also found evidence of the mistreatment of workers who were pregnant, as well as workers being prevented from using the toilet and being physically and verbally abused by their supervisors and line managers, with stories of employees being kicked and having objects thrown at them, as well as being subjected to verbal attacks. Workers even reported that agency managers would block off the factory exits to make them work overtime after their shifts had ended.[87]

Following on from the inquiry, the EHRC attempted to work with the industry to try to improve conditions. However, another investigation published in 2017 by the Bureau of Investigative Journalism revealed more cases of abuse, bullying and harassment taking place in UK slaughterhouses, with an industry source stating there was 'plenty of day-to-day abuse that is just accepted as part of the culture and environment'.[88]

A different investigation also by the Bureau of Investigative Journalism revealed that slaughterhouse workers are employed in one of the most dangerous jobs in the UK, with workers suffering from crush injuries, eye damage, amputations and loss of limbs, and even death.[89] Slaughterhouse work has also been linked to severe mental health problems.

A Brazilian study from 2012 looked at the mental health of three groups of people: workers who slaughtered birds, the slaughterhouse administration staff and university students. Students scored 10 per cent higher than the administrative staff when it came to their levels of anxiety; however, slaughterers scored 70 per cent higher for anxiety and 67 per cent higher for depression.[90] Another study found that poultry workers had an 80 per cent higher rate of depressive symptoms compared to workers from companies that weren't involved in the poultry industry.[91] Slaughterhouse workers have also been shown to suffer from alcoholism, drug abuse, sleep disturbances, destructive social consequences, suicidal thoughts, PTSD and something called perpetrator-induced traumatic syndrome, which is similar to PTSD, except it is caused by having committed violent acts oneself, instead of witnessing or being a victim of a traumatic event.

As a society, we condemn people who kill animals. If someone stabbed a dog, we would presume that they were either mentally unwell or an evil person. However, we expect people who spend upwards of 60 hours a week repetitively stabbing chickens, pigs, cows and lambs to hang up their bloody aprons at the end of the day and then just integrate back into normal society. The emotional burden of doing the work that almost nobody else wants to do because of its violent nature and doing it because you feel you have no other choice and are therefore trapped must inevitably lead to desensitisation, repression and anger for many.

Throughout this chapter, I've described witnessing many terrible things that happen to animals. They stick with you as memories that you can't quite ever shake. Sometimes they just randomly fill your head or infiltrate your dreams. And the smells and sounds are so visceral and overpowering. They stay with you just as much as what you see. If I hear the screeching of tyres, the sound reminds me of the screams of the pigs I have heard being gassed to death. What started as a leisurely walk becomes a flashback to the slaughterhouse or the farm. Those bloodcurdling screams never leave you. If I sit quietly, I can hear them reverberating around my skull as if the ghosts of those animals existed inside me, a constant reminder of the transgressions I used to commit and the violence that exists every single second of every single day. An unrelenting massacre.

But for these workers, this is their life, day in, day out. They do to thousands of animals what many of us would never want to do to even one. In the words of one ex-worker, 'I had suicidal thoughts from the guilt. I still dream about it now and I can't look at dead animals packaged up in the supermarket. And think about this as you're tucking into a roast: you didn't hear the tortured screams of those animals. You didn't see them fight with every ounce of their strength to stay alive. You didn't clean their blood from the factory floor. I did, and the guilt will haunt me forever.'[92]

ACCEPTING THE UNCOMFORTABLE TRUTH

As I stated at the beginning of this chapter, what we do to animals is really disturbing to read about, but it's important that we know what happens so that we can make informed choices. Ultimately, there is no right way to do the wrong thing and exploiting and killing animals, and causing them pain and suffering when we don't have to, is absolutely wrong. Welfare guidelines and assurance schemes are nothing more than 'humane washing' – a way to ease the conscience of the consumer in the same way that companies greenwash products to make them more appealing to those who care about the environment.

These industries realise that people hate animal cruelty, and they know that most of us would be appalled if we witnessed the standard and legal practices that take place on farms and in slaughterhouses. That's why they sell us an ideal of happy animals living wonderful lives and being killed in a compassionate and kind way. But this isn't what is happening. We're told not to worry because we have incredibly high standards and a legal system that means if anyone is caught doing anything even remotely wrong, they will be punished. This is all nonsense. It is a lie. Propaganda. There really is no such thing as a happy farm animal. We are capable of so much more.

PART TWO

PLAYING WITH FIRE

4.

OUR BEST CHANCE TO PROTECT THE PLANET

Yorkshire is often referred to as 'God's own county', mostly by the people who live there (perhaps not surprisingly). I've never really felt this county-level patriotism, and though I spent the first 18 years of my life in Yorkshire, I was never that attached to the area. That being said, I do remember travelling around the Yorkshire Dales when I was a kid and staring out of the train or car window in awe as we passed the rolling fields and hills, unravelling as far as the eye could see. I wouldn't say I was an avid rambler when I was younger – most of the time, the prospect of a day trip to the picturesque Robin Hood's Bay was met with a groan and some serious dejection – yet spending time in nature did form a significant part of my childhood. And, as I got older, I increasingly enjoyed the long hikes and regular rambling holidays to Scotland that I went on with my family.

The reason I share this is to offer an admittedly personal counterpoint to the notion that millennial vegans are all city dwellers who have never been out in nature and instead prefer to complain about issues they don't actually understand. I often find this rhetoric is used to try to discredit veganism and the rise of predominantly young people consciously reflecting on their lifestyle choices. However, it does seem rather illogical to me that my experiences in the British countryside are needed to add credibility to my overarching arguments, as geographical location neither adds to nor detracts from their validity. Whether or not you live in a city has no bearing on the objective truth of what happens in animal agriculture.

Many of us are aware that animal farming has a substantial impact on the environment, with more and more information coming out all the time, despite the misinformation spread by the animal agriculture industries. But even as far back as 2006, the United Nations released a report that stated, 'The livestock sector emerges as one of the top two or three most significant contributors to the most serious environmental problems, at every scale from local to global. The findings of this report suggest that it should be a major policy focus when dealing with problems of land degradation, climate change and air pollution, water shortage and water pollution, and loss of biodiversity.'[1] Four years later, the UN then warned that a global shift towards a vegan diet was vital to save the world from hunger, fuel poverty and the worst impacts of climate change.[2]

Despite this, now more than a decade later, there is often a reluctance to acknowledge, let alone address, both politically and socially, what the problems are and what should be done to address them. So, what is animal farming doing to our environment?

THIS NOT SO GREEN AND PLEASANT LAND

It is often said with unwavering belief that most of the British landscape is effortlessly beautiful and majestic. But there is a deep underlying problem with this. According to a Harvard Law School report, 48 per cent of the entire landmass of the UK is used for animal farming.[3] It is estimated that the land used for sheep farming alone is around 4 million hectares, which is about one sixth of the entire landmass of the UK, and yet sheep only supply around 1 per cent of our caloric intake.[4] Simply put, the amount of land used for animal farming is staggering, especially as we also import animal products from abroad, such as pig flesh from Denmark and lamb flesh from New Zealand.

In the USA, only 4 per cent of the entire landmass of the 48 contiguous states is used to grow plants directly for human consumption.[5] Beef production uses around half of agricultural land in the USA but only provides 3 per cent of the population's total caloric intake.[6] Astonishingly, the United Nations reports that 26 per cent of the world's land surface is given to grazing animals.[7]

These figures may seem enormously high, but when I cast my mind back to those experiences of travelling around the Yorkshire countryside, the fields and hills were often covered in sheep, cattle and dairy cows – huge herds and flocks as far as I could see, grazing on the fields that dominate our landscapes. It now seems absurd to me that we claim that the British countryside is beautiful when in fact so much of it is barren, a desolate landscape where the only substantial life is artificially bred or facilitated by human involvement for the sole reason of raising sentient beings for the purpose of killing them. Farmers are essentially creating an artificial and manufactured version of the environment on land that has been previously destroyed or converted. Farmers will often argue that they are essential to the environment because different species of wild animals live on their land; however, all this proves is that nature can adapt to survive, which is simply a testament to the tenacity and perseverance of those animals themselves. This is especially true when viewed alongside examples of animals coming back to land that is no longer being used for animal farming. A study on an area of land in the British uplands showed that stopping animal grazing increased the number of breeding upland bird species.[8] This argument from animal farmers also completely overlooks the reality of what is happening around us.

A recent State of Nature report compared the biodiversity intactness of the UK with that of 218 other countries around the world, ranking the UK 189th. Furthermore, 56 per cent of UK species have declined since 1970, and 25 per cent of UK mammals and nearly 50 per cent of all the birds assessed are at risk of extinction.[9] We often talk about the pervasiveness of species extinction and habitat destruction in places like South America, yet we turn a blind eye to the decimation and obliteration of life here where we live. But who can blame us for not knowing? We often hear about wildfires in the Amazon but not about the burning of peatlands in the UK to create habitats for grouse with the sole intention of hunting them. Instead, we are fed the regurgitated rhetoric of an industry that incessantly tells us that it's different here.

Until I became vegan, I never noticed the huge barns that litter the countryside, buildings that bear no markings and instead sit nestled in the landscape, conspicuous yet unconsciously ignored. These often dilapidated prisons are everywhere, with hundreds, thousands and even tens of thousands of sentient beings locked inside, not because of any wrongdoing but simply because of the species they were born into.

It seems absurd to me now that I never noticed these structures, let alone questioned what they were, even though the 1.2 billion land animals that are slaughtered every year in the UK must be found somewhere. Most of us rarely see chickens or pigs outside and yet also never question where they are or how they arrive on our plate. How can animal agriculture be so prevalent, so ubiquitous, so visible and yet so hidden, so mysterious and so unknown?

A BETTER WAY

One of the biggest issues with animal agriculture is what we get in return for such a vast amount of land usage. A huge analysis conducted by researchers at the University of Oxford reviewed 1,530 studies looking at close to 40,000 farms in 119 countries around the world and the 40 food products that represent approximately 90 per cent of all that is eaten. It looked at the main systems of farming, from factory and grass-fed to plant-based. It was considered the most comprehensive analysis ever to explore the relationship between farming and the environment, leading to it being published in the highly renowned scientific journal *Science*. The study showed that even though meat and dairy take up 83 per cent of global agricultural land, they only provide 18 per cent of global calories and 37 per cent of global protein consumption.[10] In other words, animal products are staggeringly inefficient – there is a massive disparity in the amount of resources we put into animal farming compared to what we get back. Simply put, the consumption of animal products is just not tenable in a sustainable food system.

The scale of the problem can be seen by analysing what we have lost. Deforestation is one of the most concerning environmental problems we face, and as a society we look on in horror at what is happening to rainforests all around the world without realising that the countries where we live have already been deforested and much of the damage has already been done. The UK, which used to be covered in woods and forestlands but is now just an island covered in fields, is a perfect example. Only 13 per cent of the UK is now woodlands and forests with a mere 2.5 per cent being ancient woodland.[11] Of that 13 per cent, only 7 per cent is considered to be in 'good condition',[12] and half is made up of forestry plantations that support very little biodiversity. This is much lower than the average of 44 per cent in other European countries. Huge amounts of the forests of the UK have, over time, been cleared and replaced with grass pastures to feed artificially produced, selectively bred animals, all so we can produce what is an absurdly damaging product. Such a waste – of life, of resources and of our potential to create so much more and be part of a heavily diversified and significantly more harmonious world.

And there are other examples of practices we believe to be restricted to far-flung places that have taken place closer to home. In Scotland, in the eighteenth and nineteenth centuries, the Highland Clearances saw traditional crofters forcefully displaced, their homes burned down and many even killed to allow for the introduction of sheep farming on that land – in much the same way that indigenous people are being displaced in the Amazon regions by cattle farming now.

On a positive note, the University of Oxford researchers discovered that if the world shifted to a plant-based diet, we could feed every mouth on the planet and reduce global farmland by more than 75 per cent. This is the equivalent of land the size of China, Australia, the USA and the entire European Union combined no longer being needed for agriculture.[13] Consequently, a shift towards an entirely plant-based diet would provide a huge opportunity for the restoration of not just the UK's decimated landscape and ecosystems but also areas of land all around the world that have been negatively impacted by our incredibly inefficient and destructive agricultural system.

Furthermore, through the repurposing of land currently used for pasture and cropland for animal feed, we could turn huge amounts of that land into diversified arable farmland growing crops for the sole purpose of human consumption. This could also improve the self-sufficiency of some nations, which would help reduce the environmental impact of food travel and provide jobs for farmers who used to raise animals.

For example, research into the US food system found that reconfiguring cropland from producing animal feed to entirely human-edible crops, particularly ones that promote positive health outcomes, such as fruits, vegetables and pulses, would feed an additional 350 million people compared to what the same area of land produces in the current system.[14] To put that into perspective, there are around 330 million people in the USA, meaning another nation the same size could be fed with just the cropland used to currently feed animals there. In the UK, just one third of the cropland currently used to grow animal feed could provide 62 million adults their five servings of fruits and vegetables a day for the whole year – which, incidentally, is almost the entire UK population.[15]

Of course, we don't want to change all animal farms to plant farms, as we simply don't need to use all of that land to produce food, and many animal farms are situated on land that wouldn't be suitable for arable farming anyway. However, there is something else that we can do with this land, which I'll discuss later in the chapter.

ANIMAL FARMING IS A DIRTY BUSINESS

It's not just the amount of land that is taken up by animal agriculture that adversely impacts the environment – there's also the problem of greenhouse gas emissions produced by the industry. The most problematic greenhouse gasses related to animal farming are carbon dioxide, which is produced through practices such as deforestation, the destruction of natural habitats and the damaging of soil, methane, which is produced by the digestive system of ruminant animals through the process of enteric fermentation, and nitrous oxide, which comes

THIS IS VEGAN PROPAGANDA

largely from manure and fertiliser use. It is currently estimated that animal farming accounts for somewhere between 14.5 per cent and 18 per cent of total emissions.[16] This means that animal farming is responsible for more emissions than the combined exhaust fumes produced by all global transportation, which is estimated to be around 14 per cent of the total.[17]

These figures have been questioned, with some researchers calculating that the impact of methane emissions from animals has been underestimated by 11 per cent,[18] but even if animal agriculture is responsible for around 15 per cent of the global total, this is a significant impact and highlights the urgent need to address it. Fortunately, methane's short half-life means that we would see the benefits of reducing emissions of the gas in a short space of time, making it one of the most effective things we can do to reduce global warming quickly, while at the same time buying us more time to implement means of reducing carbon levels as well. This point was re-iterated in a landmark UN report released in August 2021 that stated that countries need to make 'strong, rapid and sustained reductions' in methane emissions,[19] with one of the report's reviewers saying, 'cutting methane is the single biggest and fastest strategy for slowing down warming.'[20]

In relation to our diets, when comparing individual foods, beef results in up to 105 kilograms of greenhouse gases per 100 grams of protein, compared to tofu, which produces less than 3.5 kilograms. Even the lowest-impact beef is responsible for six times more greenhouse gases and a staggering 36 times more land usage than plant proteins such as peas.[21] Importantly, the more meat that is consumed in a country, the more emissions could be saved by switching to a plant-based diet. In the USA, for example, this has the potential to reduce food emissions by anywhere between 61 and 73 per cent.[22]

Another study that analysed 313 different feasible global food system scenarios, in which enough food could be produced to feed everyone, discovered that the highest green-house gas emissions came from the ones that included a high meat demand, especially if focused on ruminant meat and milk, and the lowest emissions were from vegan diets.[23] Furthermore, a study looking at the financial cost of the climate damage caused by agriculture revealed that organic meat had the same emission-based climate costs as conventional meat, with organic even being slightly worse in the case of beef, lamb and chicken. The study found that even the lowest-impact meat (in this case organic pork) is responsible for eight times more climate costs than the highest-impact plants (conventional oil seeds).[24]

EAT LOCAL?

But what about local animal products? Are they not more sustainable than buying plant foods from abroad? Well, not according to the science. In fact, when it comes to beef, only around 0.5 per cent of the emissions come from its transportation and for lamb it is only 2 per cent, meaning that the issue with animal farming is the farming itself.[25]

A report comparing emissions from the average diet across countries in the EU revealed that transportation was only responsible for 6 per cent of the total emissions related to diet, and when the results were broken down by food items, animal products were shown to be responsible for 83 per cent of overall emissions in the average EU diet, compared to only 17 per cent coming from plant-based foods.[26] And in the USA, a study into the impacts of food choices showed that substituting calories from red meat and dairy to plant-based alternatives for just one day a week would save 0.46 tons of CO_2 equivalent, achieving the same result as having a diet with zero food miles.[27]

All of this basically shows that when it comes to food, what we eat is significantly more important than buying local. And buying local doesn't necessarily equal more sustainable anyway. For example, a Swedish study showed that it was more environmentally friendly to buy tomatoes produced in Spain than purchasing them locally in Sweden. This is because the climate in Spain means that tomatoes can be grown in fields, rather than indoors, whereas in Sweden producing tomatoes requires the burning of fuel and uses ten times more energy.[28] All of this is to say that the idea that local equals better doesn't actually hold true. However, plant-based foods being more sustainable than animal-based foods is irrefutable.

Even though this is the case, I am still constantly confronted by the local meat argument, which has become one of the cornerstones of the marketing conducted by the animal farming industries. But the only way that buying local beef could be more sustainable than buying tofu made from soya beans grown in France is if the farming of cattle flesh and soya beans were environmentally the same to begin with and the only difference was the miles the two foods had to travel. This is obviously not the case.

One of the main reasons for the misconception that importing plant-based foods is less desirable than eating homegrown meat is the belief that our food is mainly transported via planes. While this can be the case, the overwhelming majority of food is transported via cargo boats, which produce 50 times less emissions than planes. In total, only 0.16 per cent of total food miles comes from air travel, meaning that over 99.8 per cent of food miles comes from transportation other than air.[29] When it comes to aviation, the entire industry (including freight and passenger travel) is estimated to be responsible for 2.5 per cent of total carbon dioxide emissions and 3.5 per cent of total global warming.[30]

This is why hearing farmers say that a plant-based diet is not sustainable because many plant foods are imported is incredibly frustrating. It plays on a preconception that local must be better but completely ignores the science. This isn't at all to say that food miles aren't important – they absolutely are – but reducing food miles doesn't help if doing so means eating more environmentally damaging foods.

A WALK ON THE WILD SIDE

As soon as I no longer thought of the UK countryside as a healthy environment and instead saw it for what it truly is, I began to think about the potential of what it could become. One of the major environmental benefits of shifting to a plant-based diet isn't just that it would reduce our overall emissions, it also provides us with a unique and incredibly important opportunity to do something more as well. As I mentioned previously, shifting to a plant-based diet could free up more than 75 per cent of the total agricultural land that is currently being used. As well as allowing us to produce more food in individual countries, which would be great for transitioning farmers, it would also mean we could reforest, rewild and restore a huge amount of the natural world that has been devastated by human development. This is so important because restoring the natural world will allow us to sequester carbon, which essentially means drawing carbon down from the atmosphere. If we take trees as an example, through the process of photosynthesis, they absorb CO_2 from the atmosphere and release oxygen. They then use the carbon to grow new trunks, stems and roots, thereby storing it and reducing the levels in the atmosphere.

This is one of the main reasons why a plant-based diet is one of the most important drivers of sustainability: it doesn't just remove one of the biggest contributors when it comes to greenhouse gas emissions; it also facilitates and maximises the potential for one of the best solutions to remove carbon from our atmosphere. In fact, it is estimated that if we were all to eat plant-based diets, the land no longer needed to produce food could be returned to nature and remove the equivalent of 8.1 billion metric tons of carbon dioxide from the atmosphere each year over the course of 100 years, which is about 15 per cent of the world's total greenhouse gas emissions.[31] So, not only would a plant-based diet reduce total emissions by 13 per cent, but it would also allow us to sequester a further 15 per cent of total annual carbon emissions on top of that.

The Paris Climate Agreement, a legally binding treaty on climate change that was signed by more than 190 countries back in 2015, agreed the intention of keeping global warming below two degrees Celsius above pre-industrial levels, with the aspiration to keep it below 1.5 degrees Celsius. However, a research paper from the University of Oxford showed that even if fossil fuel emissions were eliminated immediately, the emissions produced by the agricultural sector alone would make it impossible to limit warming to 1.5 degrees Celsius and would even make it difficult to keep it below two degrees.[32]

The most thorough analysis looking specifically at what dietary changes are needed in order to meet the Paris Climate Agreement combined data from every country to assess the impact of food production on the global environment. It showed that in countries such as the UK and USA, consumers need to reduce their beef, lamb and pig flesh consumption by 90 per cent and their poultry and milk consumption by 60 per cent, as well as increase their legume consumption by 500 per cent and nuts and seeds consumption by more than 400 per cent in order to keep global temperature increase under two degrees Celsius.[33] If the aspiration is 1.5 degrees, we will need to go even further. And although it's important to note that a plant-based diet won't entirely solve the problem of global warming on its own, there is also no complete solution without it.

BUT WHAT ABOUT GRASS-FED BEEF?

Another argument I hear a lot, related to the idea of carbon sequestration, is that grass-fed animals are beneficial for the environment. Animal farming proponents call these so-called environmentally friendly systems of farming 'regenerative animal farming' or 'holistic management', the basic idea being that grazing animals sequester carbon back into the soil and improve biodiversity, both of which can be true. However, the biodiversity gains are only seen when grass-fed farming is compared to intensive-farming practices. When it comes to biodiversity, the highest abundance is found in areas of unconverted land, meaning the best thing we can do is rewild and reforest farmland. As a recent UN-backed study puts it, 'The protection of land from conversion or exploitation is the most effective way of preserving biodiversity, so we need to avoid converting land for agriculture. Restoring native ecosystems on spared agricultural land offers the opportunity to increase biodiversity.'[34]

Grazing animals sequester carbon through the process of photosynthesis. When the animals graze on pasture, they consume the grass. This process then stimulates the plants to grow back and can cause their roots to grow deeper into the soil, which in turn means they sequester more carbon through the process of photosynthesis. However, this process also leads to enteric fermentation, where some of the carbon that has been eaten by the animal through the grass is turned into the greenhouse gas methane during the digestive process and is released through the animals belching. And as the cattle produce manure and urine, this creates methane and nitrous oxide. The methane and nitrous oxide are then released into the atmosphere and contribute to global warming at rates significantly more potent than carbon dioxide. So while it is true that grazing animals can sequester carbon back into the soil, the extent claimed by the animal farming industry has been refuted by the scientific literature. In fact, a team of international researchers decided to look into the claims being made and discovered that although certain grazing managements can sequester carbon, even using generous assumptions at best this could only offset 20 to 60 per cent of the emissions that would be produced by grazing the animals in the first place.[35]

The piece of research, entitled 'Grazed and Confused', also showed that after a few decades the soil reaches carbon equilibrium, meaning it cannot sequester any more carbon, at which point none of the emissions from the animals are offset. So, farmers would either have to start grazing on more land, increasing the land used for animal farming, or stop farming altogether. This means that grazing animals is not an effective short- or long-term strategy for dealing with the problem.

The Drawdown Report, a piece of research that analysed the best ways we can reduce and sequester carbon from our atmosphere, stated that plant-rich diets were four times more effective at removing carbon from the atmosphere when compared to managed grazing systems.[36] Why would we limit the amount of carbon we can sequester (especially using a system that is still a net contributor to the climate problem) when we could return agricultural lands back to nature, not only increasing biodiversity but also maximising the carbon capture potential of that land?

THE RACE AGAINST EXTINCTION

U ltimately, natural habitats, particularly forests, are able to sequester more carbon than pasturelands and would do a much better job of restoring lost biodiversity. This is so important, as species extinction and biodiversity loss are among the most urgent issues we currently face, with leading researchers saying that we are in the sixth mass extinction and facing biological annihilation.[37] In a recent red list of threatened species from the International Union for Conservation of Nature, 28,000 species were evaluated to be threatened with extinction, with agriculture and aquaculture listed as being a threat to 24,000 of them. While this doesn't mean that agriculture and aquaculture are necessarily the only threats faced by those species, it does reiterate what has already been shown: 'The consumption of animal-sourced food products by humans is one of the most powerful negative forces affecting the conservation of terrestrial ecosystems and biological diversity. Livestock production is the single largest driver of habitat loss.'[38]

An interesting argument sometimes levelled against vegans is that if we stopped breeding the animals that we eat into existence, we would make these species of animals extinct. However, the animals that we consume are selectively bred and often dependent on humans for survival because of this. The fact that they would go extinct without humans just proves that they are not natural animals to begin with. There would still be wild cattle, wild chickens and wild species of the other animals we farm; there just wouldn't be domesticated chickens whose organs fail within weeks or domesticated sheep who are unable to shed their wool. Furthermore, it seems back to front to worry about the extinction of animals who have been selectively bred and don't exist naturally to begin with when our current system of animal agriculture is the number one driver of species extinction more generally.

To see the extent of just how much animal farming has changed the biological structure of the world we live in, we need only look at the state of the world's biomass, an ecological term that refers to the total amount of living matter, including animals, plants, fungi, bacteria and other micro-organisms.

Alarmingly, one study reports that 96 per cent of mammal biomass is now just humans and farmed animals.[39] It is startling that humans only make up 0.01 per cent of the Earth's total biomass and yet we have caused the loss of 83 per cent of all wild mammals, 80 per cent of marine mammals and half of all plants. Half of the Earth's animals are thought to have been lost in the last 50 years alone. At the same time, the number of animals that we are breeding into existence keeps growing all the time. So, we are now living through a biodiversity crisis, while paradoxically creating more and more farm animals. Of course, these animals are products of years of selective breeding and artificial insemination and are not bred for the sake of the planet but instead for our dinner plates.

The problem is so immense that research published by the Royal Society has stated that animal farming has changed the global biosphere to the point where future archaeologists and historians will define our current time through the fossilised remains of the mass of farmed animals that they will find.[40]

One of the biggest problems caused by species extinction is the loss of insects and wild pollinators. It's a well-known fact that bee populations are in decline across the world, which can lead to us believing that consuming honey is beneficial for the environment. However, in the UK alone, there are around 270 bee species, with the honeybee being but one of those species. Honeybees compete directly with wild pollinators.[41] They are extremely efficient at collecting pollen and returning it to their hives but they consequently remove natural resources that are needed by the wild species. Honeybees are also significantly less effective at pollination than wild bees and other pollinators[42] but because they can out-compete wild pollinators, when honeybees are introduced into an area they can then force wild bees and other pollinators out of it,[43] which in turn makes it harder for wild plants to reproduce, further perpetuating the collapse of wild pollinators.

The Department of Zoology at Cambridge University stated:

> The crisis in global pollinator decline has been associated with one species above all, the western honeybee. Honeybees are artificially bred agricultural animals similar to livestock such as pigs and cows. But this livestock can roam beyond any enclosures to disrupt local ecosystems through competition and disease . . . Saving the honeybee does not help wildlife. Western honeybees are a commercially managed species that can actually have negative effects on their immediate environment through the massive numbers in which they are introduced.[44]

Unfortunately, while well intentioned, urban and hobby beekeeping can actually cause more harm than good. This is especially true as there are now more bee species on average in cities than in the surrounding farmlands.[45] Although many of us care about conservation and are rightfully alarmed by the demise of wild species, insects or otherwise, we are consistently missing the main driver of biodiversity loss. If we want to protect wildlife, we have to stop the destruction of wild habitats and the best way to do that is to change what's on our plates.

DEAR FARMERS, ENOUGH WITH THE GASLIGHTING

The animal agriculture industry often downplays the effect that animal farming has on the environment by making claims that on further scrutiny reveal a very significant and troubling reality. For example, the National Farmers' Union (NFU) claims that agriculture is only responsible for 10 per cent of the emissions produced in the UK and that since 1990 there has been a 16 per cent reduction in the amount of emissions produced by the agriculture sector.[46] Sounds great, right? Well, the 10 per cent figure doesn't include indirect emissions caused by animal farming, which are things like land use and land use change and often account for the majority of the animal farming industry's emissions.[47]

When it comes to the reduction in emissions, there are a couple of explanations for this decrease that are never mentioned by the NFU. First, there has been a reduction in the number of ruminant animals being farmed in the UK.[48] One of the reasons for this is that the milk yield from dairy cows has increased by around 60 per cent since 1990.[49] While this has benefits for the environment, the trade-off is the extra burden that this higher yield places on the bodies of the mother cows, who are producing significantly larger quantities of milk, which, as we've seen, puts a huge strain on their bodies and increases the incidence of mastitis,[50] a painful infection of the udders that can increase pus levels in milk and requires antibiotics to treat.[51]

Additionally, since 1990, there have been two major agricultural crises in the UK: BSE (which will be discussed in more detail in the next chapter) and foot-and-mouth disease. Both events were caused by malpractice within the farming community and resulted in the slaughter of millions of animals, reducing the overall number of cattle and sheep being farmed in the UK and imposing health regulations that created extra costs and had a long-lasting effect on the agricultural landscape that is still felt to this day. For example, in 1992 there were four million breeding ewes in Scotland, but by 2018 this had declined to 2.6 million.[52, 53] In total, the production of red and processed meat declined by almost 12 per cent in the UK between 1990 and 2018.[54] Ironically, the NFU are inadvertently making an argument in favour of veganism: if you want to reduce emissions, reduce the number of animals being farmed.

The second major reason for a reduction in emissions was due to a decrease in nitrous oxide emissions, stemming from a decline in synthetic fertiliser use.[55] This is largely thanks to an increase in the amount of animal feed that is now imported, particularly soya. The UK imports somewhere around 3.2 million tonnes of soya every single year,[56] 68 per cent of which comes from South America.[57] This soya is sourced mainly from the Amazon rainforest, the Cerrado, the Atlantic Forest and the Gran Chaco. A further 16 per cent comes from the Netherlands – but as approximately 60 per cent of soya in the Netherlands comes from South America as well and it's a re-exporting country, a significant percentage of this soya will have originally come from South America too.[58] In terms of land usage, the UK's annual demand for soya requires 1.4 million hectares,[59] meaning as many as 1 million hectares of land in South America is used to produce the UK's soya imports. Worryingly, only 20 to 30 per cent of the UK's soya is currently certified as being sustainable and deforestation free.[60]

Of this imported soya, at least 90 per cent of it is used as feed for farmed animals, with at most 10 per cent being used to feed humans directly.[61] Of the 90 per cent that is used as animal feed, the poultry industry is the number one consumer, using around half of all the imported soya to feed birds in the meat and egg industries.[62] And this usage has gone up dramatically, with a 60 per cent increase in the production of poultry flesh since 1990.[63] The next biggest user is the pig industry, followed by the aquaculture (farmed fish) and dairy industries.[64] So although we're told to support British farmers and our packets of bacon, chicken or eggs have little Union Jacks on them, there's a little piece of rainforest in almost every bite.

One of the first conversations I ever had about veganism came just shortly after I had gone vegan. I had just become aware of the environmental impact of animal farming and was relaying this information to my eco-conscious friends at university, when someone who had been listening to the conversation came over to tell me that 'soya farming is destroying the Amazon rainforest' and deforestation was on my hands because I drank soya milk. This is a common accusation that vegans face.

However, somewhere in the region of 75[65] to 80 per cent[66] of all the soya that is produced globally is used as animal feed. Looking specifically at South America, 90 per cent of soymeal produced in Brazil is used as animal feed,[67] and 96 per cent of all the soya produced in South America is used as animal feed or for cooking oil.[68] Plus, it's easy to go on to the websites of plant-based brands to find out where they source their soya from. Brands such as Alpro and Provamel, for example, only get their soya from Europe and North America.

It's not only soya that is imported to feed our farmed animals, as more than 70 per cent of the maize and rapeseed that are used as animal feed is also imported from abroad.[69] As stated by the NFU themselves, 'Many shoppers are aware of the international food chains which bring them fruit and vegetables out of season but perhaps are not aware of the feed chain behind their meat, eggs and dairy.'[70]

It's no wonder, therefore, that nitrous oxide emissions from UK farms have dropped when you consider the amount of feed being imported has increased so dramatically. As a report by the Royal Society put it, 'The UK is increasingly reliant on international trade to satisfy its food and feed demand which is accompanied by a shift in the environmental impact beyond its own territory. This is consistent with previous studies showing the impact on other environmental indicators, for example, 75 per cent of the water footprint of the UK lies overseas.'[71]

So not only have we seen a decline in production of ruminant animals, which brings down emissions from within the UK, but we have begun importing more feed from abroad, which also creates the appearance of a reduction in emissions from UK farming. The reality is that the NFU tried to claim a victory from a reduction in emissions that was caused because of two national scandals, increasing animal suffering, a lower amount of red meat production and farmers importing more feed from abroad, especially South America. This is the definition of textbook PR spin.

I can think of no other union that holds anywhere near as much power in influencing the government, and there is no better summary of this than to simply point out that the London address for the National Farmers' Union is 18 Smith Square, Westminster, London, and the address for DEFRA, the government Department for Environment, Food and Rural Affairs, is 17 Smith Square, Westminster, London. If we wouldn't trust oil companies and fossil-fuel lobby groups to be objective when discussing climate change, why would we trust the NFU, a farmer-funded membership organisation and lobby group, to be objective about animal farming?

IT'S NOT JUST BLOOD THAT'S
THICKER THAN WATER

During a televised debate I had with the chief executive of the National Sheep Association on the BBC, he referred to sheep as being the 'ultimate renewable technology'. This comment summarised to me a huge part of the problem: we have reduced the natural world and animals to simply being resources that we can do with as we please.

It's exactly this attitude that has got us into the situation we are in now. Even ignoring the fact that sheep farming is hugely damaging, our ability to look at a sentient individual and call them 'renewable' because we can just keep breeding more of their species is a perfect indictment of our mentality towards the animals we exploit. They are not even seen as individuals. By contrast, the ethics of veganism prompts us to reshape our relationship with all of the beings with whom we share this planet. As long as we view other animals as resources, we will continue to view the natural world as a resource as well. And the longer our domineering attitude continues, the graver the consequences will become, even jeopardising our ability to grow food.

Soil degradation is one of the most pressing environmental issues that we currently face, as damaged soils release carbon back into the atmosphere and diminishing soil fertility impacts our ability to grow food. Intensive agriculture in the UK has caused arable soils to lose somewhere in the region of 40 to 60 per cent of their organic carbon,[72] and globally a third of the Earth's soil is acutely degraded because of agriculture.[73]

Animal agriculture is one of the leading causes of soil erosion,[74] which can in turn lead to agricultural runoff and synthetic fertilisers and manure spreading from fields into lakes, streams and rivers. When the manure and fertilisers reach the water sources, they increase the amount of nitrogen and phosphorus in the water, which in turn causes algae to grow, creating blooms. This process is called eutrophication and could be reduced globally by 50 per cent if we stopped animal farming.[75] Algae blooms lower oxygen levels in the water, which in turn causes marine animals to die. Algae blooms further impact wildlife such as birds and mammals who eat fish for their survival. Eventually, the algae and other organisms die as they compete for the remaining oxygen and nutrients in the water. This leads to the creation of dead zones, in which most aquatic species simply cannot survive. One of the worst is in the Gulf of Mexico, where a seasonal dead zone forms every year. Its size varies from 5,000 square kilometres to 22,000 square kilometres.[76] This dead zone is blamed on the animal farming industries and in particular on companies such as Tyson Foods, who generate around 55 million tons of manure a year.[77]

Tyson Foods is the second largest polluter in the USA[78] and has been subject to multiple lawsuits for illegally dumping manure and slaughterhouse waste into waterways, even polluting drinking water in Oklahoma.[79] However, when Scott Pruitt, the Oklahoma attorney general at that time, took over the case, the judge decided to not issue a ruling on the lawsuit and Pruitt did not file an appeal either. It was later discovered by the Environmental Working Group that Pruitt had received more than $21,000 in campaign contributions from executives and lawyers at Tyson during the time of the lawsuit. In fact, almost a tenth of Pruitt's campaign contributions at that time came from agricultural sources.[80] Astoundingly, Pruitt later became the administrator for the Environmental Protection Agency, the government agency that is tasked with overseeing environmental protection matters, with one of the core purposes of the job being to enforce the nation's Clean Water Acts. Unfortunately, we simply cannot expect these industries to regulate themselves effectively or appropriately, and nor can we trust that our elected politicians are going to hold them accountable. Indeed, the only reason these industries have been able to expand and get away with everything that they do is because of the policies and allowances made by our elected governments.

In 1997, Smithfield, a meat-processing company, was found to have violated the Clean Water Act 6,900 times, spilling millions of gallons of pig manure into rivers and creeks. They were fined $12.6 million, or 0.035 per cent of their annual sales.[81] However, the worst spill occurred in 1995. A 120,000 square foot manure lagoon on a pig farm in North Carolina burst, sending more than 25 million gallons of excrement through neighbouring fields, over a road and into the New River. Within just a couple of hours, dead fish began to line the riverbanks, and within a day they were covered. The manure was so viscous it took two months to travel sixteen miles along the river and downstream to the ocean, killing everything along the way. In total, it is conservatively estimated that 10 million fish died and 350,000 coastal acres of habitat were polluted.

But this was just the beginning of the problem. After the spill, millions more fish developed large bleeding sores before suddenly dying, and fishermen along the river experienced severe respiratory problems, headaches, and visual and mental impairment, with some forgetting how to get home. The spill had created *Pfiesteria*, a microbe that can bloom from the nutrient-rich waste from pig farms. In total, *Pfisteria* has killed a billion fish in the USA. However, Smithfield and other meat, dairy and egg companies are able to act with relative impunity and are never held properly accountable for the damage that they cause.

It's not just the USA that has a major problem with water pollution. The UK has the worst bathing water quality in Europe,[82] with only 14 per cent of the rivers in England being of a good ecological standard,[83] and no river having a good chemical status.[84] This means that every river in the country is contaminated with harmful pollutants. Farming is reportedly the largest contributor to severe water pollution, with dairy farming causing the highest number of serious incidents.[85] In fact, the areas of Wales that have seen their sea trout population collapse almost precisely overlap with the locations of dairy farms, with reportedly only 1 per cent of farm slurry stores (slurry is a mix of water and manure used as fertiliser) in Wales meeting regulations.[86]

An Environment Agency investigation also revealed that 95 per cent of farmers around the River Axe in southwest England have inadequate slurry containment facilities that do not comply with regulations, with 49 per cent of them consequently polluting the river.[87] Yet, despite this, in 2015 the UK government attempted to reduce the number of farm inspections and overhaul the greening requirements that farmers had to meet to be able to receive the EU farming subsidy.[88] They even wanted to reduce the number of inspections to check ecological focus areas, which are areas of land where farmers are meant to carry out practices that are beneficial for the environment and biodiversity. In the same year, the government even bragged that they had 'cut 10,000 unnecessary dairy inspections a year' since 2010.[89] This deregulation isn't even happening behind closed doors; it's openly discussed and celebrated by the farming industries and the government alike. Meanwhile, the quality of our water continues to get worse.

The River Wye, which is the fourth longest river in the UK and has been designated as a Special Area of Conservation and encompasses two Sites of Special Scientific Interest

(SSSI), has also become increasingly polluted, with an increasing number of areas becoming prone to algae blooms, the culprit in this instance being free-range poultry farms. The chicken excrement gets spread on the ground around the sheds and is then flushed into the river, causing plants and fish to die off. Even when farms are documented as having violated the rules, they never receive a punishment. Between April 2018 and the start of 2021, there were 243 documented violations (even though this is estimated to be a fraction of the actual number). Not a single one of those violations resulted in prosecution or even a fine.[90]

To add insult to injury, 150 new intensive poultry units have been approved for the area around the River Wye in the past five years alone.[91] More farms, more pollution, more algae blooms, more dead zones and a further eroding of the rivers and our natural world. And water pollution isn't the only issue when it comes to animal farming. Droughts are becoming an increasingly more prevalent issue globally and it has even been theorised that the wars of the future will be over water. Needless to say, freshwater is a huge concern, both from an environmental perspective and also a humanitarian perspective. Animal farming accounts for around a third of the world's freshwater consumption[92] with animal products requiring more water to produce than crop products.[93] In fact, a meat-free diet can reduce an individual's water use by as much as 58 per cent.[94] If we want to conserve our water, going vegan is a big step in the right direction.

DON'T TEACH A MAN TO FISH

Alongside agricultural runoff, the fishing industry is one of the other major contributors to the creation of these marine dead zones, with 415 such areas having been identified worldwide.[95] The Baltic Sea is home to many of the world's largest, with the overfishing of cod in particular being highlighted as one of the main causes.[96]

The fishing industry contributes to other environmental problems in the oceans as well. Somewhere between 50 to 80 per cent of all the oxygen production on Earth comes from photosynthesis by bacteria and marine phytoplankton – tiny ocean plants.[97] The oceans also absorb 25 to 40 per cent of all carbon dioxide emissions[98, 99] and play a pivotal role in regulating temperature and overall climate, which isn't really surprising, considering that around 70 per cent of the Earth's surface is covered in water.[100]

As we have seen, the two main methods of catching wild fish are bottom trawling and longline fishing. Bottom trawling is a particularly popular method in commercial fishing because it can catch large quantities of fish in one go. However, when dragging the large, weighted nets across the seafloor, everything that happens to be in the way gets swept up in the net too, leading to huge amounts of unwanted fish, known as bycatch, and damage of the seafloor, which also helps to create harmful algae blooms and oxygen-deficient dead zones.

In addition, bottom trawling has been shown to produce as much as 1,500 million tonnes of CO_2 each year, which means this fishing method produces more emissions on average than the entire aviation industry.[101] These emissions are due to marine sediments, the largest global carbon store, becoming displaced and releasing carbon as a result of the trawling. However, commercial fishing is also responsible for releasing carbon into the atmosphere through the removal of marine animals from the ocean. Phytoplankton, which as previously stated absorb carbon, are then eaten by sea animals who often go on to be eaten by even bigger sea animals. When terrestrial organisms die, they release carbon into the atmosphere as they decompose; however, marine animals sink deep into the ocean when they die, which means that most of the carbon released from their bodies can be sequestered and stored. This carbon is referred to as 'fish carbon', and because we remove somewhere in the region of 0.8 to 2.3 trillion marine animals every year from the oceans, we are taking fish carbon out of the oceans, with part of this then being stored in the atmosphere instead. In the same way that restoring terrestrial ecosystems provides us with a great opportunity to sequester carbon, the same is true with restoring our oceanic ecosystems as well.

For example, before industrial whaling severely reduced the whale population, scientists estimate that as much as 1.9 million tonnes of carbon could have been sunk into the ocean annually through whales alone, which is equivalent to removing 410,000 cars off the road each year.[102] It has been estimated that rebuilding the population of just large baleen whales would provide the equivalent carbon capture potential of 272,000 acres of forest, an area the size of the Rocky Mountain National Park.[103]

The benefit of healthy whale populations goes beyond even this, as whale excrement contains iron and nitrogen, two nutrients that phytoplankton need to grow. In effect, the migration of whales leads to the fertilisation of the ocean and subsequent increase in phytoplankton, which can then sequester carbon. The International Monetary Fund (IMF) estimates that just a 1 per cent increase in phytoplankton would be the equivalent of adding two billion mature trees to the world.[104] In other words, having healthy oceans that are filled with an abundance of life is essential to a sustainable planet. Unfortunately, our oceans are far from being healthy.

Longline fishing is the other commonly used method of catching fish; it is estimated that there is enough long line set every day to wrap around the planet 500 times.[105] Similar to bottom trawling, the lines are indiscriminate, meaning that bycatch is also a huge issue. Every year, around 650,000 whales, dolphins, seals, sea lions and turtles are killed because of the fishing industry[106] – the equivalent of more than one every minute. On top of that, it is estimated that 100 million sharks are killed each year, either for their fins through illegal fishing or unintentionally as bycatch.[107]

It is also estimated that 10 per cent of all fish caught are discarded,[108] which means many species are being fished to the brink of extinction simply as an unintended consequence of commercial activities, which is in turn having a big impact on the biodiversity of the oceans. In fact, around 90 per cent of the world's fish stocks are now fully fished or overfished.[109] To make matters worse, 20 per cent of wild fish that are caught are fed to farmed animals, including farmed fish but also pigs and chickens,[110] meaning our oceans are being destroyed to feed animals in an industry that is further contributing to environmental degradation in a whole host of other ways – such as greenhouse gas emissions, habitat destruction, deforestation and pollution.

The damage caused to marine life and habitats by the amount of plastic in the ocean has come to particular public attention in recent years. It is reported that as much as 70 per cent of macroplastics found floating on the surface of the ocean is fishing related.[111] A recent study of the 'Great Pacific garbage patch', an area of plastic accumulation in the North Pacific, showed that 86 per cent of the macroplastics in this area were fishing nets.[112] Furthermore, discarded fishing nets are the most deadly form of plastic pollution, posing the greatest risk to marine life.[113]

Aquaculture now provides more than half of all the fish that are consumed globally,[114] but the problems caused by this industry are intrinsically linked with those of wild fishing. This is because many of the fish raised on farms are carnivores, so they need to eat smaller fish to live. Billions of wild fish are therefore caught in order to feed these farmed species. There is also the issue of crops being used for feed as well. For example, a review study showed that for every 19 grams of protein from eating farmed fish, around 100 grams of protein will have been fed to the fish, and for every 10 calories we get from farmed fish, 100 calories will have been used in their feed.[115]

One of the biggest issues related to fish farming is the high emissions it produces, with even the lowest-impact aquaculture systems producing more emissions than vegetable proteins.[116] Perhaps surprisingly, the highest-impact farmed fish can produce even more emissions than beef.[117] This can be due to a number of factors, such as clearing carbon sinks like mangroves to make space for the farms, the energy that is used to operate the pumps and regulate temperatures for farms that are not in the sea and the production of feed, as well as excrement and unconsumed feed dropping to the bottom of fish ponds and producing methane and nitrous oxide.[118] Farmed fish are also a leading cause of algae blooms and water pollution.[119] Furthermore, the high rates of disease in fish farms, including sea lice, have a negative effect on wild fish populations as well. The wild salmon migrate past the sea pens containing the farm salmon and become infected with the lice. A review study showed that sea lice from fish farms can lead to a 29 per cent reduction in adult wild salmon, with wild sea trout mortality levels expected to be even higher.[120]

There has been some good news. In July 2021, Argentina became the first country in the world to ban salmon farming because of concerns about their environmental impact. Let's hope other countries follow suit as well.

A SUSTAINABLE FUTURE IS A VEGAN FUTURE

All of these problems – such as water pollution, the rise in greenhouse gasses, the drastic reduction in biodiversity – have come about on a planet with just under eight billion people on it. Within the next 30 years, our population is expected to increase to 10 billion.[121] However, global trends show that food consumption isn't increasing proportionally to the growing population but rather regardless of the increase in population. This means that overall food demand is predicted to be 50 per cent higher by 2050, with animal-based foods being 70 per cent higher and specifically ruminant meat being 88 per cent higher.[122] An additional 593 million hectares of land will be needed to meet this demand, which is nearly the equivalent size of two Indias.[123] This will mean more deforestation and land conversion, more habitat loss and species extinction, more freshwater use, more soil erosion and more greenhouse gas emissions. Simply put, we can't afford to keep animal product consumption at the levels it is at currently, let alone increase consumption by 70 per cent.

Something clearly has to change. Shifting to a plant-based diet is one of the most significant decisions that we can make as individuals to reduce our impact on the planet, and moving to a plant-based food system that also focuses on reducing food waste needs to be an essential part of sustainability goals. It provides us with the best opportunity possible to reclaim huge expanses of land that can be reforested, rewilded and restored, improving biodiversity, sequestering carbon and significantly reducing, among other things, water pollution, agricultural emissions, soil erosion, species extinction, habitat destruction and deforestation. In the words of the lead author of the most comprehensive analysis on farming and the environment to date, who incidentally started his research as a meat eater but became vegan because of the findings of the study, 'A vegan diet is probably the single biggest way to reduce your impact on planet Earth, not just greenhouse gases, but global acidification, eutrophication, land use and water use.'[124] Going vegan really is our best chance to save the planet.

5.

VEGANISM COULD SAVE
YOUR LIFE

I remember watching a news report in the mid 2000s about the spread of bird flu around the world. It featured a map of the world with images of birds superimposed over the countries that were battling outbreaks of bird flu. As the reporter described how the outbreak was spreading, the images of the birds began moving towards the UK. Being only 12 or so years old, I didn't really understand what was being reported and had little understanding of the potential impact of an influenza outbreak, but I remember feeling an ominous sense of dread that this was an issue of real concern.

The prospect of a pandemic is incredibly frightening. Not only can they kill millions of people, but they can cause so much suffering in the process. Infectious disease is in many ways the ultimate existential threat. Unlike the climate crisis, which we've been warned about for decades, infectious diseases can arise at any moment and, within the blink of an eye, change the world as we know it. In recent history, the question around pandemics has been *when* there will be another one and not *if*. However, the inextricable link between our exploitation of animals and the creation and spread of infectious diseases is often overlooked. If we want to ensure that the issue of pandemics is not simply a question of when, we have no choice but to stop exploiting animals.

THE UNPRECEDENTED RATE OF EMERGING DISEASES

I f there is one thing I'm sure most of us don't want to hear about ever again, it's Covid-19. And yet the most dangerous thing we could do now is to pretend that it never happened. That's the approach we have taken many times before, but, as we keep learning, infectious zoonotic diseases (originating from non-human animals), epidemics and even pandemics will not go away by us simply carrying on as though it is business as usual.

Unfortunately, we have a history of being dangerously complacent about the possibility of infectious disease. In fact, in 1948, US Secretary of State George Marshall declared that the conquest of all infectious diseases was imminent.[1] Sadly, this turned out to be nothing more than wishful thinking, with the World Health Organization (WHO) declaring almost 60 years after this statement was originally made that 'new diseases are emerging at an unprecedented rate'.[2] The organisation subsequently tracked 1,483 epidemic events in 172 countries from 2011 to 2018 alone.[3]

Even though Covid-19 has been a devastating pandemic, resulting in the deaths of millions of people and costing trillions of dollars, leading infectious disease experts and scientists have still referred to it as a dress rehearsal.[4] A senior WHO official declared that the Covid-19 pandemic should be a 'wake-up call' but warned that it is 'not necessarily the big one',[5] a term used to describe the category five pandemic that experts dread. For reference, Covid-19 is a category two pandemic.[6, 7]

Whenever there is an outbreak of a deadly disease that is effective at human-to-human transmission, containment will always be an incredibly difficult task, especially in a modern world with global travel and densely populated cities. Consequently, the key to pandemic and infectious-disease prevention is stopping these diseases from emerging in the first place. But to do that we have to understand what causes them.

It is estimated that about 75 per cent of new or emerging infectious diseases in people come from non-human animals,[8] meaning that our relationship with other animals is of the utmost importance when trying to reduce the risk of infectious disease. Animal farming in particular has been linked to an increasing list of outbreaks and diseases. Back in 2004, the WHO, the World Organisation for Animal Health (OIE) and the United Nations Food and Agriculture Organization (FAO) released a joint report in which they listed rising demand for animal protein as being the first point on their list of the biggest risk factors in the creation of infectious zoonotic disease.[9] Since then, the same message has been continuously emphasised by a number of organisations. In 2013, the FAO reiterated their deep concern when they stated that 'livestock health is the weakest link in our global health chain'.[10]

So why is it that taking a bite out of an animal could in turn come back to bite us as well?

Coronaviruses

On 30 December 2019, Ai Fen, the director of emergency care at Wuhan Central Hospital, received the lab results from a patient she had seen with flu-like symptoms. The results read 'SARS coronavirus'. (The Latin word *corona* means crown, because under a microscope the virus has a crown-like appearance.) Before the twenty-first century, coronaviruses had caused infectious-disease experts little concern, as the known coronaviruses that affected humans at that time were responsible for causing only mild illnesses, such as the common cold. However, that all changed in 2002 when an outbreak of SARS (severe acute respiratory syndrome) began in the Guangdong Province in China. The outbreak wasn't just a freak occurrence.

Throughout the 1990s, the trade in wild animals for both food and supposed medicine grew rapidly in China due to the expanding middle class and economic transformation that was taking place. This led to the farming of wild animals becoming increasingly intensive, with large numbers of animals being raised in cramped conditions and transported, often over borders from different countries, to live animal markets. In these markets, dozens of species of animals mix; their blood, saliva, urine and faeces contaminate floors, tables and other animals, and all in an environment filled with humans, often in densely populated cities. It was these conditions that provided a perfect opportunity for the first truly deadly coronavirus to emerge.

Scientists strongly believe that SARS started as a virus in bats before then being passed to civet cats,[11] who served as an intermediary host in which the virus could mutate and become capable of animal-to-human and then human-to-human transmission. Interestingly, although the genetic building blocks for the virus originated in bats, without the civet cat link, the virus might never have gained the ability to lock onto the enzyme coating the cells of human lungs.[12] In other words, the outbreak occurred because of the mixing that was enabled by live animal markets and the wildlife trade in general. In response to the outbreak, the Chinese government initially enacted a ban on the trade of civet cats, but within months that ban had been lifted.

SARS ended up infecting 8,096 people, killing 774 of them.[13] Thankfully, it never became a pandemic, largely due to the fact that it always resulted in a fever and human carriers weren't contagious until they started to exhibit symptoms, and even then the infectiousness of the virus remained low for the first several days of the illness. This meant that robust screenings at airports and self-isolation were able to stop the virus from spreading effectively. The worrying thing was, though, that SARS had a fatality rate of just under 10 per cent and transformed our perception of coronaviruses from little more than an inconvenience to potential full-blown mass killers.

A decade later, in 2012, the next outbreak of a deadly coronavirus occurred, this time referred to as MERS (Middle East respiratory syndrome). The intermediary hosts on this occasion were camels, which had been domesticated thousands of years previously. So, what had changed to facilitate the emergence of MERS? The increasing numbers of overgrazing camels in the Middle East had led to a lack of habitat and resources, so the camel industry had begun to shift to high-density enclosed systems of farming and housing, creating more close contact between camels and humans.[14] In Qatar, the country with the highest camel density in the Middle East, open grazing of camels was banned in 2011, which led to a significant number of camel workers and owners crossing the border to and from Saudi Arabia.[15] One year later, the first case of MERS was identified in Saudi Arabia.[16]

MERS is even more deadly than SARS, killing 858 of the 2,494 humans it has infected so far, meaning it has a fatality rate of around 35 per cent.[17] Again, thankfully, the outbreak didn't escalate into something much worse, due to the virus requiring close contact for effective animal-to-human and human-to-human transmission. Unfortunately, the camel industry's PR campaign 'Kiss Your Camel', which was created in response to the Saudi Arabian government's advice to avoid contact with camels and the consumption of camel flesh and milk, and which was meant to deflect blame for the virus away from camel farming, encouraged probably the least advisable action for a virus that spreads to humans who have close contact with the respiratory system of the animals.[18]

It was because of these two epidemics that when Ai Fen received the results from the tests she had run, she sent the information to other leading doctors, spreading the message that an outbreak of coronavirus was underway. As we all now know, this outbreak was triggered by a novel coronavirus, one that was fortunately not as lethal as both SARS and MERS, but was, unfortunately, much more infectious.

The first known outbreak of this virus was in the Huanan market, which reportedly sold dozens of different wild species, including mammals who, judging from the fact they had wounds from gunshots and traps, appeared to have been caught illegally from the wild.[19] When environmental samples were taken at the market, over 90 per cent of those that were positive for Covid-19 were found in the section that was selling exotic and wild animals for food.[20]

While it is still not definitely known which species acted as an intermediary this time, one theory is that it could have been pangolins, who are also the most trafficked mammal in the world, killed for their meat and scales.[21] However, it may be some time before we know for sure, as scientists weren't able to prove that civet cats were the intermediary species for SARS until early 2007, over four years after the epidemic began.[22] It also took until 2017 for scientists to find samples from bats that had all the essential genetic building blocks that make up the human SARS virus that had caused the epidemic.[23]

However, the animal that many infectious disease experts fear the most is not a wild or exotic species; it is, in fact, the land animal that is most exploited around the world.

Influenza

To most of us, flu consists of a fever, cough, sore throat and body aches. However, in 1918 the flu meant something much worse. The 1918 pandemic, sometimes referred to as the 'Purple Death', is the most severe pandemic in recorded history – it killed 50 to 100 million people and infected one third of the world over a period of two years.[24] Although the symptoms were familiar in the early stages of infection, as the virus took hold millions died from internal bleeding, choking on blood and pus, organ rupture and in other horrific ways. Pockets of air accumulated under sufferers' skin due to ruptured lungs, causing them to crackle as they turned over, and purple blood blisters appeared, hence the name Purple Death.

Unlike Covid-19, fatalities in the 1918 pandemic weren't largely elderly people; in fact, quite the opposite – it disproportionately killed younger people, with the average age of death being 28.[25] The virus killed so many people that it actually brought down the US average life expectancy by 12 years.[26] Survivors recall how cities ran out of caskets, with dead bodies left to rot and mass graves having to be dug. Homeless children wandered the streets, orphaned when their parents were killed by the virus.

But what caused it? At the time of the pandemic, little was known about infectious disease and influenza viruses, meaning that for decades there were still many unanswered questions about the origins of the virus. In 1997, in the search for answers, the pathologist Johan Hultin travelled to the tiny Alaskan city of Brevig Mission, where a postal carrier had spread the virus to the small city during the pandemic, killing

72 of the 80 missionaries who lived there. The remaining missionaries subsequently buried the dead in a mass grave.

Among the skeletons in the mass grave, the body of a woman, who Hultin called Lucy, was discovered whose internal organs had been preserved by the cold climate, meaning her lungs could be taken to be studied. This revealed that the 1918 pandemic was caused by a strain of avian influenza. This discovery was groundbreaking in our understanding of the evolution of influenza and has importantly helped define what can be done to reduce the risk of such a pandemic happening again.

It is now strongly believed that all influenza A viruses (the type of influenza viruses that have pandemic potential) originate from birds and that the spread of flu from birds to humans first occurred due to the domestication of ducks about 4,500 years ago.[27] In fact, the domestication of animals in general combined with humans becoming less nomadic and settling in communities triggered a mass spillover of many animal diseases into human populations. Unsurprisingly, many animals who live in groups are prone to contagious diseases due to the fact that the viruses can spread easily between hosts; however, it is also these herd animals that were most suitable for domestication, which meant bringing many of these diseases into sustained close quarters with humans for the first time. As a result, diseases such as tuberculosis, measles, whooping cough, diphtheria, smallpox, influenza,[28] the cold virus,[29] and the list goes on, are thought to have originated from the domestication of animals, with more spillover events happening all the time.

The spread of disease during the colonisation of North America and genocide of Native Americans at the hands of European settlers illustrates the pivotal role that domestication had on the spread of disease. Before colonisation, there were essentially no epidemic diseases in the Americas[30] – and there were no domesticated animals either.[31] While pockets of disease and outbreaks will have occurred, as they would have among nomadic humans in Afro-Eurasia as well, the absence of close, sustained contact between animals and humans meant that spillover events of diseases like tuberculosis, measles and the flu had simply not happened. When Europeans began to colonise, they brought with them domesticated animals and, as a result, diseases for which Native Americans had no immunity. In total, Native American death rates from diseases such as the flu and smallpox ranged by region from 33 per cent to as much as 90 per cent.[32]

But how did influenza become a deadly disease for humans? In its original form, influenza has existed for millions of years as an intestinal waterborne infection in aquatic birds. The virus survived by spreading in the lakes and ponds that the birds frequented, being excreted into the water by the waterfowl and then passing to the other birds who were also using the water. The influenza virus didn't make the animals sick, because it didn't need to in order to survive and spread; in fact, the birds displaying their natural healthy behaviours was beneficial for the spread of the virus. In essence, the virus had evolved to exist in a form of harmony with its hosts.

Aquatic bird influenza has not historically caused serious disease or harm to humans, with only a handful of medically recorded reports of people being infected with the aquatic wild bird virus, which only caused a mild case of conjunctivitis.[33] Scientists have also attempted to actively infect humans with the aquatic wild bird influenza virus but failed to get it to take hold of the human volunteers, even with very high doses.[34] This of course makes sense – the gut of a duck, where the virus resides, is after all very different to the lung of a human. So what changed?

With the domestication of animals, the relationship between multiple species drastically altered. All of a sudden, water

VEGANISM COULD SAVE YOUR LIFE

birds were mixing with terrestrial birds such as chickens, who were not natural hosts but were genetically similar enough to become infected by the virus as well. However, because the virus was no longer able to spread in the manner it had done for millions of years, via the water used communally by large numbers of aquatic birds, it was forced to adapt to be able to survive. And so while mutations in the virus in aquatic birds never took hold, in their new hosts mutations began to change the genetics of the virus, allowing it to spread to different organs of the body, such as the lungs.

Once the ducks were able to pass the virus on to chickens and to domesticated pigs, the animals acted as mixing vessels for the virus, allowing it to mutate, going through a process called reassortment. This meant it could lock in the necessary genetic mutations required to then jump into humans and be effective at binding to our receptors.

After a virus has infected a new host, it is confronted with an immune response that it has not encountered before. Met with this immune response, the virus is forced to fight for its survival, and in doing so it can become deadly to its host. However, being too deadly doesn't always work advantageously for the virus; if it wipes out its host too quickly, it limits how effectively it can spread, thereby jeopardising the ability of that particular mutation to survive. This is why many viruses can become less deadly over time: the process of natural selection works to find the point of relative harmony between a virus and its host that best allows the virus to survive and spread – the sweet spot of lethality and contagion. This is also why the influenza virus has evolved to target the lungs in humans, as it is able to take over the cells, reconfiguring them to make them produce more virus, which helps the virus spread within the body while at the same triggering an inflammatory response in the lungs that causes a cough. The virus essentially hijacks the body's defence systems to facilitate its spread to other humans.

In the case of the 1918 pandemic, the most comprehensive analyses that have been conducted to find its origins point to it beginning in the USA, initially spreading between the Camp Funston military facility in Kansas and Haskell County, Kansas.[35] It is thought that there was a comparatively mild first wave of the virus there during the early spring of 1918, with the first recorded cases occurring at Camp Funston. Reports stated that Haskell County smelled of manure because of the poultry, cattle and pig farms that were there and at Camp Funston, pigs and poultry were kept at the camp and the soldiers were housed in overcrowded accommodation, providing the perfect opportunity for a spillover event to take place and the virus to spread efficiently.[36] It then travelled across the Midwest with the troops as they crossed the country on trains, visiting cities on the way before boarding transport ships and heading to Europe.

Later that year, the virus mutated into a killer, taking advantage of the fact that it could achieve its full lethality and contagion potential due to the unusual conditions created by the First World War. It spread through the crowded environments the soldiers were living in, with the uninfected unable to avoid or escape those who were sick. This meant that killing off its hosts too quickly was less of a disadvantage than is usual, as the virus had access to hundreds of thousands of potential hosts who were immunocompromised, some suffering respiratory problems due to the effects of noxious gases used in the war and many having weakened immune systems as a result of stress and lack of good nutrition. Then, once the war ended, the virus was able to travel around the globe as the troops returned home. And so a virus that was first recorded in a military camp in the USA went on to kill 50 to 100 million people around the world.

It would seem on the face of it like the risk of a similar pandemic is small, especially considering it's highly unlikely we will ever replicate the conditions of the First World War. And yet the same kind of environment that facilitated the spread of the 1918 virus now exists all over the world. Not on the Western Front, but instead in every intensive pig, chicken and egg-laying hen farm, with millions of animals crammed into tiny, unhygienic, enclosed spaces, immunocompromised and unable to escape from the sick or dying animals around them. We've recreated the trenches of the First World War with our farm animals – not forgetting the people who work with them every day – and the global transport industry can now do an even better job of spreading a virus to all corners of the world than the troops returning to their many home countries and states after the war ended did. In addition, we've gone one better by creating genetically uniform animals through the selective breeding process, which further allows infectious diseases to spread. In the case of broiler chickens, their accelerated growth rate weakens their immune systems, making them especially susceptible to disease.

Following the 1918 pandemic, there were two further avian influenza pandemics in the twentieth century and a swine influenza pandemic in 2009. Thankfully, none of them were as severe as the 1918 pandemic, but the 2009 swine flu was yet another reminder that we are always playing catch up when it comes to our knowledge of influenza viruses. The 1918 pandemic was an H1N1 bird flu virus, which, as well as being passed on by humans, also infected pigs. In fact, the 1918 pandemic was the first time pigs were known to have been infected with influenza,[37] although it is possible that it had gone unnoticed before then. After the pandemic ended, a reassortment of the virus turned into swine flu and another reassortment became the regular seasonal flu for humans.

After a couple of near misses in the 1950s and 60s, something that had never happened before took place in the late 1990s. In North Carolina, a state renowned for its huge number of pig farms, the swine flu virus combined with the circulating human flu and a bird flu to create a triple-animal reassortment virus. The virus was then spread around the country by the long-distance journeys that pigs go on as they are transported to different farms and slaughterhouses. By 2005, the virus began to spill over more frequently into pig farm workers, before eventually causing the 2009 swine flu pandemic.[38] It is estimated that somewhere between 150,000 and 575,000 people died worldwide as a result, with 80 per cent of those deaths occurring in people younger than 65.[39] However, infectious disease experts had been fearing something much worse.

In 1997, the worst fears of infectious disease experts came close to being realised. Thousands of chickens began dying in Hong Kong, their faces turning black and their bodies shaking as they died, often by choking on large blood clots that were blocking off their airways. When autopsies were carried out, it was discovered that the chickens' internal organs had been reduced to bloody pulp. A couple of months later, in May of that year, a three-year-old boy was the first human to be admitted to hospital with the virus, where he died from multiple organ failure and his blood having curdled. Tests revealed that he had died from a new strain of avian influenza, H5N1.

The second human to die was a 13-year-old girl, whose lungs and intestines haemorrhaged and whose kidneys failed. Disturbingly, the virus was shown not just to affect the lungs but to target other organs as well, even attacking people's brains and causing fatal comas.[40] This widespread infection throughout the body was something that even the 1918 virus wasn't capable of.

Sadly, more cases of H5N1 soon occurred, causing panic among the medical and scientific communities. Once the origin of the illness was traced back to chickens, leading scientists called for every chicken in the entire Hong Kong area to be culled, which they were, and the spread of the disease was subsequently stopped. In total, eighteen people were infected and six died. Fortunately, the virus wasn't effective at human-to-human transmission and so was unable to spread efficiently. However, this wasn't the end of H5N1. The virus arose again in the early twenty-first century and began killing humans in 2003, at which point it spread from Hong Kong and travelled across Asia, emerging in eight countries simultaneously, due to the wide transportation of chickens in the region.

Hundreds of millions of birds were culled. Horrendous methods were employed, such as the animals being burned and buried alive, but this didn't stop the virus, which continued to spread into the Middle East, Africa and Europe. Since its first emergence in 1997, the virus had been mutating, reassorting many times and becoming more accomplished at spreading. H5N1 even began to infect and kill animals such as pet cats, who had never been recorded as suffering from the flu until H5N1.[41]

To date, H5N1 has infected 861 people and killed 455.[42] Terrifyingly, this means it has a fatality rate of around 60 per cent, but thankfully it has still not acquired the necessary mutation to make it effective at human-to-human transmission, although that could happen at any moment. Every time there is a spillover, there is a risk that the virus has locked in the necessary requirements to spread in the same way that the seasonal flu does, and if that were to happen, we would be dealing with a virus that would make Covid-19 look insignificant in comparison. H5N1 is a virus that can kill anyone, regardless of age or health. Put into perspective, the 1918 pandemic had an estimated fatality rate of somewhere around 2.5 per cent.[43]

If this virus ever did mutate to have pandemic potential, it is likely that it wouldn't retain its horrifically high 60 per cent fatality rate, but even more modest estimates still predict it could have somewhere between a 14 and 33 per cent fatality rate,[44] making it anywhere between 5.5 and 13 times worse than the 1918 pandemic, which was the most severe pandemic in recorded history. The fear is that in the modern world, where the virus resides in animals who are crammed together in barns or on farms, and are in direct contact with humans and regularly transported through cities to slaughterhouses and wet markets, before coming into contact with people who live in densely populated cities and are able to move around easily thanks to constant global air travel, the virus is far less limited by its ability to spread – all it has to do is lock in the right mutations and we'll do the rest. The prospect of anything more severe than the 1918 pandemic is almost too horrific to think about and yet, while we continue as we are, with the expansion of animal farming and our growing population, the risk grows alongside us.

And if a pandemic of this severity were to occur, it wouldn't just be the deaths the virus caused that we would need to be concerned about. We got a glimpse of what panic can do to people at the start of the Covid-19 pandemic when people fought over toilet roll and stockpiled food. What would happen if there were genuine food shortages or there weren't enough doctors and nurses to treat patients because they were dying or were too afraid to come to work? It wouldn't just be the infected who died but those being treated for other illnesses such as cancer, or those who had heart attacks or strokes but couldn't call an ambulance. What would happen if utilities like internet, water and electricity were affected?

All of this may seem hyperbolic, but the events of the Covid-19 pandemic would have seemed unlikely to most of us before they happened, and the reality is the only reason we have escaped an H5N1 pandemic so far is because of luck. And yet at any point we might be unlucky. The virus might spill over once again, but this time with the mutation to make it as contagious as Covid-19.

Following the 1983 H5N2 bird-flu outbreak in Pennsylvania that resulted in the culling of 17 million chickens, US poultry farmers began to use antivirals in the water supplies at their farms, even though doing so creates drug-resistant mutations,[45] rendering antivirals that can treat viruses completely useless to humans in the event of one of these resistant strains spilling over. And all to reduce economic loss from bird flu deaths among the birds. Much to the horror of the world, this is exactly what happened in 2005, when an exposé revealed that Chinese poultry farmers had been giving antiviral drugs to their chickens, meaning that H5N1 had become completely resistant to them.[46]

However, it's not just H5N1 that poses a risk; in fact, the influenza strain ranked by the Influenza Risk Assessment tool developed by the Centers for Disease Control and Prevention (CDC) in the USA as having the greatest potential to cause a pandemic, as well as posing the greatest risk to public health, is H7N9,[47] a virus that has so far infected 1,568 people, killing at least 616, meaning it has a fatality rate of around 40 per cent.[48] Again, thankfully, the virus has still not gained effective human-to-human transmission. Worryingly, though, there are influenza outbreaks happening all the time, including in poultry farms,[49, 50] and we have even seen human infections, one as recently as June 2021.[51]

When it comes to outbreaks of infectious disease, it is easy to point the finger and place the blame on other countries and cultures, something that became very evident at the beginning of the Covid-19 pandemic. However, the risk of infectious disease isn't restricted to Asia, or even to wet markets – though it is worth noting that wet markets also exist in the USA, with more than 80 in New York City alone, and bird flu viruses have been found there.[52] Between 1959 and 2015, the majority of conversions of low-pathogenic avian influenzas – strains that pose a low risk of illness and death to chickens and little threat to human health – to highly pathogenic avian influenzas – strains that pose a high risk of illness and death to chickens and a much greater threat to human health – have occurred in Europe and the Americas.[53] In the USA, between December 2014 and June 2015, highly pathogenic avian influenza was reported in 242 premises, leading to 50 million farmed birds being killed.[54]

We have created a system of agriculture that means we intensively farm tens of billions of birds and pigs every year – animals who are mixing vessels to take diseases that carry almost no risk to humans and turn them into mass killers that could cause the deaths of hundreds of millions of people. As the WHO stated in a report about avian influenza, 'Highly pathogenic viruses have no natural reservoir. Instead, they emerge by mutation when a virus, carried in its mild form by a wild bird, is introduced to poultry. Once in poultry, the previously stable virus begins to evolve rapidly, and can mutate, over an unpredictable period of time, into a highly lethal version of the same initially mild strain.'[55]

Ultimately, we can't rely on the poultry industry to safeguard us, especially when it is their constant priority to make what they do more cost effective that has caused so many of these problems in the first place. However, there is one important aspect of current infectious disease control that we should take note of. Whenever there is an outbreak, every bird who could be infected is culled – it was this strategy that stopped the spread of H5N1 back in 1997. So, the current method of control already acknowledges the most important aspect of pandemic prevention: when you remove the animals, you remove the risk.

By continuously breeding and farming animals, we are putting ourselves in a position where we are forced to be reactive.

But all it takes is one slip-up, one spillover event that we can't control, and hundreds of millions of people could die. If we stopped eating poultry products, we could eliminate the part of the process that turns avian influenza into a mass killer, and because the overwhelming majority of chickens are killed at around six weeks, within two months we would have all but eliminated the biggest threat in the creation of highly pathogenic avian influenza. Stop eating pigs and within six months we would have all but eliminated the next biggest influenza threat.

When you consider the enormity of suffering and death that could be caused by an influenza pandemic, the farming of animals is clearly incredibly dangerous, not to mention needless. Although we might not think about how a bite out of a chicken burger could negatively impact the world in such a profound way, the reality is that our desire for meat could well be what brings our civilisation to an end. So, while we may enjoy the taste of chicken and bacon, I'm sure we can all agree that we like our organs not being reduced to a bloody pulp, our lungs being able to breathe and millions of people not dying from a preventable pandemic even more.

Deforestation and Bushmeat

It's not just the environments in which the animals are kept that makes livestock farming responsible for increasing the risk of spillovers; the acquisition of land for farming requires habitat loss and deforestation. This is especially problematic in tropical areas of the world where disease-carrying animals and insects such as mosquitos, rodents and bats, among others, can be found.

A novel disease in India that had a 5 per cent fatality rate was linked back to a tick-borne monkey virus, the origin of which was traced to the clearance of forests for cattle grazing.[56] In Brazil, malaria cases have been recorded to be steadily rising in parallel with forest clearing for the expansion of agriculture,[57] the vast majority of which is for animal farming.[58] The Junin virus in Argentina and Machupo virus in Bolivia are both driven by human agricultural activities,[59] mainly animal farming.[60, 61] The spread of yellow fever in Brazil has been linked to increased deforestation[62] – the biggest culprit is, once more, animal agriculture.[63] Then there's Nipah, a disease that has a fatality rate as high as 75 per cent.[64] This was caused by the clearing of forests for agriculture in Malaysia that forced fruit bats to look elsewhere for food. They found trees around one of the biggest pig farms in the country, which led to half-eaten fruit from the bats being consumed by the farmed pigs, causing an outbreak among pig farmers.[65]

It is of course important to mention that agriculture is not the only reason for deforestation and increasing contact with wild animals – the logging and mining industries also substantially contribute to the problem; however, the biggest driver of land use and deforestation is animal agriculture, with 41 per cent of global tropical deforestation being caused by cattle farming alone.[66]

Then there is Ebola, a truly horrifying disease that can cause internal haemorrhaging and has an average case fatality rate of 50 per cent.[67] The 2014 to 2016 outbreak, which is the worst outbreak of Ebola so far recorded, infected more than 28,000 people and killed in excess of 11,000.[68] It is believed to have originated from the consumption of wild animals, often referred to as bushmeat.[69] It's a similar story for HIV, a disease that is strongly believed to have originated from the butchering and consumption of chimpanzees.[70] Tragically, more than 30 million people have died from AIDS-related illnesses since the start of the epidemic, and to this day a person dies from an AIDS-related illness every minute.[71]

The issues related to bushmeat, though, are of course very different to those posed by industrial farming. If we all stopped eating poultry and pork, we would remove the two biggest risk factors in the creation of influenza pandemics, but there are other factors at play when it comes to bushmeat consumption. Most of us eat meat because we like it, not because we have to; however, for many people in lower-income nations, the consumption of bushmeat is a necessity. A 2016 report highlighted how Chinese and European-subsidised fishing vessels were contributing to decreased fish populations in the coastal regions of West Africa, forcing more people to turn to bushmeat for food, which in turn increased the risk of Ebola outbreaks.[72] In essence, our consumption of fish is creating food scarcity for those in low-income nations. So, as well as being a contributing factor to previous Ebola outbreaks, it could also be the cause of the next one.

There is of course a difference between subsistence hunting and the commercial bushmeat trade, much of which has been made illegal by many countries in Africa. Unfortunately, in the same way that meat-eating in Western countries is seen as a status symbol, the same is true of bushmeat in African nations, where for many its consumption is a cultural practice.[73] Because of the cultural aspect of eating bushmeat, large quantities are smuggled out of Africa; it's been estimated that as much as five tonnes of illegal African bushmeat is brought into Europe each week via Charles de Gaulle Airport in Paris alone.[74] Some of this bushmeat is then sold at markets such as the one in Ridley Road in London, where an investigation by the BBC in 2012 found smuggled bushmeat for sale.[75] Another investigation two years later revealed that illegal meat was still being sold at the same market.[76] Bushmeat has also been found on sale in other cities across Europe[77] and in the USA.[78]

It's not just dead animals that pose a risk in the spread of infectious disease, though; the trade, both legal and illegal, of live animals also creates the potential for disease to spread. The SARS and Covid-19 outbreaks are two good examples, as is the aforementioned Nipah outbreak, which was only able to spread so efficiently around Malaysia and into Singapore because of the transportation of live pigs.[79] The first reported outbreak of the Marburg virus in 1967 took place in Marburg, Frankfurt and Belgrade, and killed 70 of the 31 people it infected. The outbreak was traced back to the importation of African green monkeys from Uganda for animal testing and research.[80]

The international trade of exotic pets, a highly lucrative industry worth billions of dollars, also poses a substantial risk.[81] In 2003, an outbreak of monkeypox virus in the USA was traced back to the importation of 800 small mammals into Texas from Ghana.[82] In the UK, in 2005, finches imported from Taiwan for the pet trade were discovered to be infected with H5N1.[83] Fortunately, they were in a quarantine facility, so the disease could be contained, but the illegal trafficking of wild animals and pets is an ever-growing concern when it comes to the spread of infectious disease, especially as it bypasses any regulated quarantine facilities.

BSE

I grew up in the aftermath of the BSE (bovine spongiform encephalopathy) crisis. Even though I was too young to remember the crisis itself, growing up I still saw the images of piles of dead cows being incinerated and videos of cows struggling to walk, and I was aware of the ill-fated government mantra that 'beef is safe to eat'. The BSE crisis showed us that nowhere is immune to the dangers of animal farming and that these issues can start close to home, too. But how exactly did BSE come to exist?

On 22 December 1984, a cow on a UK farm named 'number 133' developed head tremors and a loss of coordination. Two months later, she was dead.[84] At the same time, other cows began to show similar symptoms. BSE, also referred to as 'mad cow disease', which slowly destroys the brain and spinal cord of cattle and is always fatal, officially became recognised as a new disease in 1986, albeit confidentially.[85] However, because the UK government didn't ban bovine offal (the cattle parts that could be contaminated) from being used in human food until the end of 1989, this meant that they knew that BSE-infected beef was potentially entering the food supply chain for several years.

It is strongly believed that BSE was created because farmers were feeding cattle meat-and-bone meal, which is the rendered remains of animal flesh that is considered not suitable for human consumption. The meat-and-bone meal contained the ground-up remains of other ruminants, including cattle and sheep, which has led to the theory that BSE could have been triggered by cattle eating sheep infected with scrapie,[86] a neurological disease. Or it could have resulted from a genetic mutation in cattle in the 1970s.[87] Either way, the disease then spread further by the rendered remains of BSE-infected cattle being fed to more cattle. Farmers and feed companies were forcing herbivorous animals to cannibalise simply because it was the cheapest way to feed them.

As the number of cases began to increase, the UK government slaughtered millions of cattle, with 4.4 million being culled in total.[88] Unsurprisingly, the British public became increasingly worried that they could be infected by eating beef. So, in 1990, the agriculture minister John Gummer attempted to feed his daughter a beef burger in front of the British press to alleviate people's fears. She shied away from the burger, so he took a big bite instead, declaring it 'absolutely delicious'.[89] Unfortunately, five years later, on

21 May 1995, 19-year-old Stephen Churchill became the first known human to die from variant Creutzfeldt–Jakob disease (vCJD). However, initially his death was listed as being caused by classic CJD, a pre-existing rare neurological disease, with the UK government even going so far as to continue to emphasise that British beef was safe to eat and refusing to carry out an inquiry into his death, even though there was concern Stephen Churchill's death was related to the BSE crisis.[90] Numerous dairy farmers had also been diagnosed with and died from classic CJD leading up to Stephen Churchill's death, but the UK government was adamant there was no link to BSE, even though behind the scenes there was growing unease, so it was never discovered whether or not it was the BSE-related vCJD that was the actual cause of their deaths.[91] In 1996, the British government eventually backtracked and declared that the consumption of BSE-infected cow flesh had in fact created a new disease called vCJD.[92] However, by this point the damage had been done. Nobody knew just how much infected flesh had been eaten.

Similar to BSE in cows, vCJD causes neurological decline. Symptoms include hallucinations; loss of speech, bladder control and movement; blindness; confusion; and eventually death. It is a disease that wouldn't have existed if it weren't for the actions of the farming industry. As of 2015, there have been 229 known cases of vCJD and 229 deaths.[93]

Worryingly, according to the *Lancet*, there is now evidence that vCJD can lie dormant for more than 50 years.[94] A study in the *British Medical Journal* showed that as many as one in 2,000 people in the UK may be carriers of the abnormal protein that is associated with the disease,[95] meaning the worst of the crisis for humans may yet be to come. The impact might even be beginning to be felt now, as the rate of classic CJD cases diagnosed has doubled since the mid

1990s.[96] However, most of these people were not given autopsies, meaning there's no way of knowing if it is the variant caused by BSE or not. Additionally, as stated in a report published by the UK government, there is evidence that cases of classic CJD and vCJD could be misdiagnosed as Alzheimer's disease.[97] A leading expert from the Association of British Neurologists went so far as to state that there could be 'massive under-ascertainment' in the diagnosing of classic CJD and vCJD.[98] This all means that there could be a silent epidemic happening right now.

Thankfully, it is now illegal to feed ruminant animals the rendered remains of other ruminant animals. However, it is still legal in the UK for blood products to be fed to non-ruminant animals, such as pigs and chickens.[99] In the USA, poultry litter, which is essentially a mixture of feathers, excrement, spilled feed and birds who have died on the farms, can be used as animal feed, including for ruminants. This means that poultry litter used as feed for cattle could still contain the rendered remains of other cattle, as it can include spilled poultry feed, made from cows.[100]

Back in 1996, Gary Weber, who was the director of beef safety and cattle health for the National Cattlemen's Association, defended the practice of forcing cattle to cannibalise by saying, 'Now keep in mind, before you view the ruminant animal, the cow, as simply a vegetarian – remember that they drink milk.'[101] Ridiculous, nonsensical statements such as these hardly inspire confidence in the beef industry's willingness or ability to take this issue seriously.

Foodborne Pathogens

Infectious diseases that arise from our food chain and have the potential to seriously threaten our health are not limited to viruses that mutate and become epidemics and even pandemics. They can also be found in supermarket fridges all the time – they could even be in your fridge right now.

The scale of disease and contamination in our food supply is so vast and normalised that we often don't even realise that there is a problem at all. In total, it is estimated that there are 2.4 million cases of foodborne illness in the UK each year.[102] For example, nearly three quarters of chickens sold in supermarkets and butchers is contaminated with campylobacter – a bacteria that can cause vomiting, diarrhoea, fever and even death – with 19 per cent being 'heavily contaminated'. It is even present on 7 per cent of packaging tested.[103] In total, around 280,000 people in the UK are made ill by it every year, with around 100 people dying as a result.[104] The scale of the problem is so significant that in 2014 the Food Standards Agency (FSA) even considered publishing the names of supermarkets and chicken producers and their campylobacter rates to push them to improve. However, the proposal was initially voted down, with Tim Bennett, the former president of the National Farmers' Union, also voting in favour of protecting chicken producers.[105]

A year later, the FSA did publish the findings of a year-long testing programme that revealed the rates of campylobacter, even though the UK government unbelievably attempted to pressure the FSA into not publishing them. The government, alongside the poultry industry, was actively trying to hide information from consumers that would have allowed them to avoid buying food that was infested with this potentially fatal bacteria. Not only that, but if the government had succeeded, it would have removed pressure on chicken producers to improve, instead leaving them to self-regulate without any fear of public accountability.

This became painfully apparent in 2018, when an undercover investigation was carried out into a 2 Sisters Food Group factory in West Bromwich,[106] which is the largest supplier of chicken flesh to UK supermarkets and produces one third of all poultry products eaten in the UK.

The investigation discovered that the workers there, under instruction from supervisors, had tampered with food safety records, which could have led to consumers being duped into buying flesh that was past its use-by date by switching labels. The investigation also revealed that workers had altered the records of where chickens were slaughtered, which is extremely dangerous, as it makes it difficult to recall flesh if there is an issue with food contamination or disease.

On top of this, chickens that had been returned by supermarkets were being repackaged and then sent out again with new use-by dates. This was documented happening with chickens who had been packed for the supermarket Lidl but were then returned to the processing facility by the retailer. They were then repackaged with pieces of other chickens for Tesco and labelled with the name of one of Tesco's fake promotional farms, called 'Willow Farms', with the statement that the contents of the pack are 'reared exclusively for Tesco'.

It's a similar problem in the USA, where the CDC estimates that around 48 million people get sick from a foodborne illness each year.[107] Testing has shown that 60 per cent of pork products, 70 per cent of beef, 80 per cent of chicken products and 90 per cent of turkey products are contaminated with E. coli.[108] Simply put, faecal contamination is a huge problem for the meat industry, especially as animals in slaughterhouses often defecate because of the fear they feel. The problem is so common that poultry officials in the USA considered using superglue to seal the anuses of birds in slaughterhouses so that there would be less risk of contamination.[109] But even if such a gruesome practice was ever implemented, it wouldn't stop the spread of excrement when the birds are cut up and their organs pulled out, which can cause the rupturing of the intestines. Chickens are also often plumped as well, a process in which they are soaked or tumbled in water to increase their weight. As soon as the soaking water is contaminated, it can spread to all the other chickens being plumped in the same water – the water is sometimes referred to as 'fecal soup'.[110]

But even abstaining from eating animal products doesn't necessarily safeguard you from the problem, as is evident from outbreaks of E. coli linked to the consumption of lettuce, spinach and other plants. In fact, between 2005 and 2020, there were 40 E. coli outbreaks linked to contaminated lettuce in the USA alone.[111] But plants don't have intestinal systems, so how are they becoming contaminated? Because of manure spreading and water contamination from nearby animal farms. Unfortunately, not even plant foods can escape the disease created by animal farming.

Antibiotic Resistance

Any bacterial issues we face right now will pale in comparison to what the WHO has described as one of the biggest threats to global health.[112] Unfortunately, as soon the animal farming industries realised that giving antibiotics to farmed animals not only decreased mortality rates but also acted as a growth promoter, the writing was on the wall.

In 1951, the US Food and Drug Administration (FDA) approved penicillin and tetracycline for animal use, and within just a couple of years the same practice was being adopted all around Europe, with many different types of antibiotics being used.[113] Medicated feeds became omnipresent in the poultry industry, with the rise of intensive farming largely facilitated through the mass use of antibiotics. By the end of the 1950s, the same thing was happening in pig farms, and by the mid 1960s it was estimated that 80 per cent of mixed feeds for pigs, veal calves and poultry in Germany contained antibiotics.[114] They were even being used by Norwegian and Icelandic whaling vessels, which incorporated antibiotics into explosive harpoons to preserve the whale meat.[115] By 1970, the use of antibiotics for non-medicinal reasons, such as growth promotion, had increased by more than 30-fold in the USA; in Europe it was a similar story.

In the 1980s, experts reiterated what Alexander Fleming, the discoverer of penicillin, had warned back in 1945 when he had stated that the overuse of antibiotics could lead to 'mutant forms' that would be completely resistant to the drugs.[116] However, despite increasing concern, the growth of global antibiotic use in animal farming continued, which was matched by the growth of antimicrobial resistance. For example, seven years after the FDA approved the use of the antibiotic fluoroquinolones for use in poultry farming in 1995, bacterial resistance to the drug had increased from practically zero to 18 per cent.[117] Fluoroquinolones are classified by the WHO as being 'critically important in human medicine'[118] due to their ability to treat E. coli, salmonella and campylobacter. In essence, the poultry industry is contributing to the creation of antibiotic-resistant strains of a bacteria that consumers then catch from eating poultry. In fact, a study from the European Centre for Disease Prevention and Control showed that 60 per cent of human campylobacter cases in EU countries were resistant to ciprofloxacin, a type of fluoroquinolone, with 62 per cent of poultry infected with campylobacter carrying the resistant strain.[119] Between 2015 and 2019, UK pig farms also doubled their use of aminoglycosides, a class of antibiotics the WHO has deemed to be 'critically important' for human health.[120]

While some progress has been made in reducing antibiotic use in farmed animals, such as the EU ban on antibiotics as growth promoters, their use is still unfortunately rampant. In 2016, industry figures revealed that UK farmers had increased their use of fluoroquinolones, which are now banned in the USA, by 59 per cent in 12 months.[121] Globally, antibiotics are still routinely given out as growth promoters, including in countries such as the USA, Australia, New Zealand and Canada,[122] with an estimated 70 to 80 per cent of all antibiotics being used in farmed animals.[123] The so-called 'antibiotic of last resort', colistin, which is only meant to be used in extreme cases, has also been documented as being used on farms.[124] The miracle of modern medicine is being squandered every day, wasted so that animal production can be more cost effective. All around us, bacteria are gradually adapting, causing antibiotics to become less and less effective, until we are left with diseases that we are unable to treat.

Currently, around 700,000 people around the world die each year due to antibiotic-resistant diseases, with 230,000 of those deaths coming from drug-resistant tuberculosis.[125] The problem is so severe that even urinary-tract infections (UTIs) and sexually transmitted diseases (STDs) are becoming resistant to treatment.

If antibiotic-resistant diseases continue to increase due to the overuse of antibiotics in animal farming, we could find ourselves in a situation whereby people with cancer would have to decide whether or not it was worth having chemotherapy, as there would be a risk that they could develop bacterial infections for which there was no treatment. In essence, the choice would be: do I want to die from the cancer or from the resistant bacteria? Routine procedures like dental treatments and hip replacements could become life threatening, and pneumonia could kill millions. A world without usable antibiotics is a world where the infections and diseases we currently regard as being trivial could become deadly. Right now, it is estimated that antibiotic resistance will kill 10 million people each year by 2050.[126] To put that into perspective, the WHO has stated that cancer killed an estimated 9.6 million people in 2018.[127]

Thankfully, overall, antibiotic use in farmed animals has dropped in the UK in the past half a decade, but globally it's a different story, and, when it comes down to it, any antibiotic use on farms is a waste because of the simple fact that animal farming is completely unnecessary. The number of antibiotics that should be used to keep animals alive just long enough so we can kill them is precisely zero. In the end, we have to decide what we value as being most important: ensuring antibiotics are effective at treating our illnesses or wasting them so we can buy cheap animal products in the supermarket. I know which option I would choose – what about you?

WHEN DOES ENOUGH BECOME ENOUGH?

We have created what can only be described as the most absurd and dangerously short-sighted system of food production possible – a system that is one of the main contributors to the degradation of the planet, causes immense suffering, is squandering the most important medicines that we have and is creating viruses that cause pandemics and could even result in the deaths of hundreds of millions of people. At what point do we acknowledge how ridiculous this is? If we experience another pandemic like the one in 1918? When people have to choose between cancer or resistant bacteria? If an H5N1 pandemic happens, will we still say veganism is extreme?

In 2020, the United Nations Environment Programme (UNEP) listed the seven factors caused by humans that are driving the emergence of zoonotic diseases:[128]

1. Increasing human demand for animal protein.
2. Unsustainable agricultural intensification and in particular domestic livestock farming.
3. Increased use and exploitation of wildlife.

4. Unsustainable utilisation of natural resources accelerated by urbanisation, land use change and extractive industries.
5. Increased travel and transportation.
6. Changes in food supply driven by increased demand for animal source food, new markets for wildlife food and agricultural intensification.
7. Climate change.

Of the seven drivers listed by the UNEP, six are either substantially or entirely linked to our exploitation of non-human animals. While it is true that the risk of infectious disease spillovers will never be entirely eliminated, our current system of food production and treatment of animals in general is greatly heightening the risk and needlessly causing the emergence of highly dangerous strains of viruses and drug-resistant bacteria alike. Our approach to pandemic and epidemic prevention so far has been to cross our fingers and simply hope for the best, because, in reality, the way that we treat the natural world and animals right now is more in alignment with pursuing the maximisation of disease than it is the prevention of global health disasters.

We often claim that eating meat is a personal choice, but not only does that statement ignore the impact our consumption of animal products has on the animals themselves, it also ignores the environmental damage and the potential for deadly pandemics caused by diseases transmitted from animals raised for slaughter. While buying animal products in a supermarket might at face value seem to be a fairly innocuous decision, the far-reaching consequences are, without exception, inescapable. In essence, our everyday choices in the food that we choose to eat create a ripple effect that is felt globally. Veganism is the only way we can make sure that those seemingly innocuous decisions don't become ones we regret.

6.

THE HEALTHY CHOICE

Whenever a vegan falls ill, non-vegans always blame it on their diet. Have a cold? It's because you're vegan. Stomach bug? It's because you're vegan. Are you looking tired today? It's because you're vegan. Someone even once told me that several work colleagues in their office had come down with the flu but that when they also got it, they were told by co-workers that it must have been because they were vegan.

When I first went vegan, I too was warned about the dangers of not getting enough nutrients. Another student on the same university course as me even stated that there wouldn't be any vegan options available at the event we were organising together because 'if people don't eat meat, they'll all be fainting'. Needless to say, there is a lot of scrutiny around the healthfulness of plant-based diets. My own personal experience is of having more energy, better skin, better digestion and an increased feeling of wellbeing since going vegan – but what does the science say?

In 2009, the Academy of Nutrition and Dietetics in the USA (formerly called the American Dietetic Association), the largest body of diet and nutrition professionals in the country, released a statement regarding the healthfulness of plant-based diets:

It is the position of the American Dietetic Association that appropriately planned vegetarian diets, including total vegetarian or vegan diets, are healthful, nutritionally adequate, and may provide health benefits in the prevention and treatment of certain diseases. Well-planned vegetarian diets are appropriate for individuals during all stages of the life cycle, including pregnancy, lactation, infancy, childhood, and adolescence, and for athletes.[1]

The British Dietetic Association concurs, stating, 'Well-planned plant-based diets can support healthy living at every age and life-stage.'[2] This position is also supported by the NHS: 'With good planning and an understanding of what makes up a healthy, balanced vegan diet, you can get all the nutrients your body needs.'[3] And the same position is taken by Harvard Medical School,[4] the Mayo Clinic,[5] Dietitians of Canada[6] and many more.

Outside of the confirmation that eating a plant-based diet can be healthy, and even beneficial in the prevention of certain diseases, it's important to note that these statements emphasise the importance of a plant-based diet being well planned and balanced. The truth is, you can be a healthy vegan or an unhealthy vegan – the latter is especially true thanks to the ever-growing range of vegan burgers, 'chicken' pieces and ice creams. However, while it's good to highlight the importance of a healthy plant-based diet, it creates the impression that if you eat animal products you don't need to think about what you consume or know anything about what makes up a balanced diet, which is not true. For instance, it is estimated that only 5 per cent of US citizens are consuming the recommended amount of fibre a day, even though eating fibre-rich foods is associated with better gut health, lower cholesterol and reduced risk of strokes, heart attacks, type 2 diabetes and some forms of cancer.[7] In the UK, fewer than 10 per cent are consuming enough.[8] Around half of the US population is estimated to consume less than the recommended amount of magnesium from food, with research showing that as many as 30 per cent of people in affluent countries may have subclinical magnesium deficiency.[9] And the list goes on. The point is, regardless of whether you are eating a plant-based diet or not, it is important to know where you are getting your nutrients from and to take ownership of your own health, as anyone eating any diet can miss out on the things their body needs to be healthy.

Personally, I have found the added scrutiny on the healthfulness of a plant-based diet to be beneficial, as it has encouraged me to do proper research, take charge and make sure that I am obtaining the necessary nutrients. Before I was vegan, I had no idea what vitamin B12 was, or non-haem iron. In fact, I knew almost nothing about what foods gave me which nutrients and what I needed to be healthy. The extent of my knowledge was that vitamin C comes from oranges, calcium comes from cow's milk, protein comes from meat and omega-3 comes from fish. Beyond that, I never considered that I could be deficient or lacking nutrients in my diet. I was told that eating meat, dairy and eggs was all part of a balanced diet, so why would I need to worry?

This is a huge part of the problem: we are taught almost nothing about nutrition, and a huge amount of our perception about food is subsequently created by advertising and marketing, carried out by companies who are trying to sell us something. It's no wonder we believe that cow's milk is the best source of calcium when for millions of people the 'Got Milk' campaign in the USA was a part of popular culture, with celebrities being featured with 'milk moustaches' telling us milk is an important part of a healthy diet. It was so influential that it is well recognised around the world. Milk moustaches were then used to promote dairy in the UK as well, with the 'Make Mine Milk' promotional campaign.

That animal products constitute part of a 'balanced diet' is an idea consistently perpetuated by the animal farming industries. An advert promoting red meat and dairy consumption that was screened on UK televisions in early 2021 with the tagline 'eat balanced'[10] is a good case in point. However, this creates a false notion that if you don't eat red meat and dairy, you must not be eating a balanced diet and are unhealthy. It's a wonderful stroke of good fortune that a balanced diet just so happens to involve eating the animal products that the farmers who promote that idea want to sell you. According to this narrative, a balanced diet doesn't involve eating the flesh and secretions of other animals that are eaten around the world – such as camels, dogs, cats, whales, dolphins, horses, guinea pigs, crocodiles, kangaroos, shark fins, turtles, iguanas, monkeys, emus, and so on. Luckily for us, out of the literally thousands of edible animals that we could consume, it's the four or five animals that have been farmed where we live for hundreds of years, long before we even knew about nutrients, that are the ones important for a 'balanced diet'.

Thankfully, there are more scientifically robust recommendations of what really constitutes a balanced diet available. The EAT-*Lancet* planetary health diet is the first full scientific review of what would constitute a healthy diet within a sustainable food system. It was created by an international commission made up of leading scientists from 16 countries and published in the *Lancet*, one of the most respected medical journals in the world. It recommended that people in Western countries eat between 77 and 84 per cent less red meat, categorised eggs, poultry and dairy as optional, and confirmed that a plant-based diet is a healthy option.[11]

In response, a member of the Meat Advisory Panel said that 'encouraging people to eat less red meat and dairy will have little impact on the environment and is potentially damaging to people's health'.[12] It's frightening that such a detailed report, one that has been referred to as 'the most advanced ever conducted',[13] can be so easily disregarded by those within the animal farming industries, especially considering they have nothing even remotely comparable in terms of scientific validity or scale to support their response.

Geographical life expectancy rates don't support the position taken by the Meat Advisory Panel either. There are five areas of the world that are referred to as the 'Blue Zones'. In these places, people live exceptionally long lives, and there are comparatively very high numbers of centenarians. One of the things most notable about those living in Blue Zones is that they eat a diet that is 95 per cent plant-based.[14]

HOW TO THRIVE ON A PLANT-BASED DIET

So, while we know that you can be healthy on a vegan diet, there are some nutrients to be especially aware of to ensure we get them from plant-based sources. The first thing to note is that a healthy plant-based diet should be a wholefoods one – which means a diet centred around minimally processed plants, such as fruits, vegetables, wholegrains, pulses, nuts, seeds and legumes. Although processed vegan alternatives like meat-free burgers don't contain many of the harmful aspects of animal products and have been associated with having lower cardiovascular risk factors when compared to red-meat burgers,[15] as well as increasing the health of the gut microbiome when compared to animal products,[16] they are not the healthiest foods. So, though you can absolutely enjoy the variety of plant-based alternatives that are now available, a diet made up mainly of wholefoods is the best way to be healthy and thrive on a plant-based diet.

Protein

The question of where to source protein from will, I have no doubt, bring a smile to the face of most vegans, because even though protein is not something vegans need to be especially concerned about, we are constantly asked if we get enough of it. Protein is made up of amino acids, nine of which are considered essential, meaning they must be acquired through diet. All of the essential amino acids our bodies need can be found in plants, with some plants such as soya (which includes foods such as tofu, tempeh, soya milk and edamame), quinoa and buckwheat being 'complete' sources of protein, meaning they contain all the essential amino acids. However, you can get all the essential amino acids through food combinations as well, such as rice and beans, hummus and pita bread or a wholewheat peanut butter sandwich. You don't need to consume all the essential amino acids at the same time as long as you eat a variety of good plant-based protein sources throughout the day.

It is generally recommended that most adults eat about 0.75 to 0.8 grams of protein per day per kilogram of body weight, which on average means about 46 grams for a woman and 56 grams for a man.[17] If you work out, are pregnant or do challenging physical work, you'll need to consume a bit more. Obtaining protein on a vegan diet is very easy, and as long as you're eating the recommended number of calories for your lifestyle and body, and are making sure to incorporate some protein-rich plant foods, then you'll be fine.

Healthy sources of plant-based protein include:

- Legumes, such as beans, soy, lentils and chickpeas
- Wholegrains, such as oats, farro, brown rice and wholewheat pasta
- Nuts and seeds
- Vegetables, such as broccoli, green peas, Brussels sprouts and asparagus
- Seitan

Swapping from animal protein to plant protein has also been associated with a lower risk of premature death. In 2020, a study was published for which researchers had followed 400,000 participants aged 50 or older who consumed protein from either plant sources, red meat or eggs for 16 years. The data revealed that those who ate predominantly plant protein had a 13 to 15 per cent lower overall risk of mortality when compared to those consuming red meat and a 24 per cent lower risk when compared to those eating eggs, even when factors such as smoking, diabetes, vitamin supplementation and more were factored in.[18]

In a review of 32 studies about protein intake that included more than 715,000 participants who were followed for periods ranging from three and a half years all the way to more than 30 years, plant-protein consumption was associated with an 8 per cent lower risk of all-cause mortality, and in the case of mortality from heart disease there was a 12 per cent lower risk. The authors of the review concluded, 'These findings have important public health implications as intake of plant protein can be increased relatively easily by replacing animal protein and could have a large effect on longevity.'[19]

Although it is often believed that a plant-based diet will inhibit muscle growth, one study found that when comparing protein intake from animals or plants for muscle mass and strength, there was no significant difference.[20] In fact, studies that examined the bones of Roman gladiators showed that they primarily ate plants, especially wheat and barley, with there being little sign of meat or dairy products in their diets.[21] This fits with the name 'barley men', which was a contemporary term used to describe gladiators. There are vegan bodybuilders and strongmen, such as the Olympic weightlifter Kendrick Farris and Patrik Baboumian, a strength athlete who holds the world record for heaviest yoke (a bar or frame that goes behind the head and across the shoulders) carried over ten metres.

There are also many high-profile vegan athletes, such as Dotsie Bausch, who is an eight-time US national cycling champion, a two-time Pan American gold medallist and an Olympic silver medallist. NBA basketball stars such as Chris Paul and Kyrie Irving say that a plant-based diet increased their energy and performance levels, and there are vegan world-record-holding ultra-marathon runners, footballers and NFL players. Tennis stars Novak Djokovic and Venus Williams have both promoted the benefits of a plant-based diet, as has the Formula One driver Lewis Hamilton.

In other words, not only is getting enough protein from a plant-based diet not a problem for the everyday person, it isn't a problem for elite athletes either. They have been shown to thrive on plant-based diets and even increase their performance levels and become more successful.

Iron

Iron is an essential mineral that, among other things, helps maintain healthy blood. In particular, the body uses iron to create haemoglobin and myoglobin, which carry oxygen. In days gone by, doctors would recommend that their patients drink Guinness after surgery or giving blood. Although I am all for a nice plant-based alcoholic beverage from time to time, I wouldn't recommend stout as a good source of iron as it only contains about 0.3 milligrams per pint.

There are two main forms of dietary iron: haem and non-haem. Haem iron is only found in animal products, while non-haem iron mainly comes from plant foods. Haem iron is more easily absorbed but the body is unable to regulate its take-up, meaning that it can't remove excess amounts. This can be problematic as iron is a pro-oxidant – too much of it can lead to inflammation. Haem-iron consumption has also been associated with an increased risk of colon cancer, with one analysis associating haem-iron intake with an 18 per cent increase in colon cancer risk.[22] Clinical trials have also shown that haem iron can increase the formation of compounds[23] that can damage the cells of the bowel lining, increasing the risk of cancer.[24] And in another analysis, higher dietary haem iron intake was associated with an increased risk of cardiovascular disease, while there was no association found with non-haem iron intake.[25]

Although less easily absorbed, non-haem iron from plant foods is better regulated by the body and is often full of anti-oxidants. And combining it with vitamin C can mean it is absorbed more effectively, which can be achieved simply by squeezing some lemon over your food. Many fruits, particularly citrus fruits and berries, contain abundant vitamin C, and it's also found in vegetables, where it is often coupled with a good source of iron to begin with, as is the case for vegetables like broccoli and kale.

It is recommended that men over the age of 19 and women over the age of 50 should get 8.7 milligrams of iron a day and women aged 19 to 50 should get 14.8 milligrams.[26] Healthy sources of plant-based iron include:

- Seeds, such as pumpkin, chia, flax and hemp
- Soya, including tofu and tempeh
- Wholegrains, such as quinoa, oats and wholegrain bread
- Nuts, such as cashews and almonds
- Legumes, such as beans, chickpeas and lentils
- Leafy green vegetables
- Dried herbs, such as thyme and parsley
- Dried fruits, such as apricots, dates and prunes

Calcium

I consider myself lucky to have avoided the free-milk-in-schools era. I always disliked the taste of cow's milk and found it deeply unpleasant to consume. I can distinctly remember my dad giving me a glass of milk to drink when I was young. It was a gesture that came from a caring place but the fact that I can so vividly recall the experience probably indicates how I felt about it. I also remember being repulsed by the smell of porridge being made because of how the milk smelled when it was being cooked (realising that oats are delicious when made with a plant milk has been a real revelation for me).

As mentioned in an earlier chapter, free milk was given to school kids and has for a long time been thought of as an essential part of a healthy diet. But this perception, which still persists today, is hugely due to the prolific marketing of the dairy industry, which has made calcium synonymous with dairy products. But while they do provide calcium, they are by no means the only or healthiest source. For example, dairy consumption has been associated with prostate cancer, as was shown in an analysis of 47 studies, incorporating more than 1 million participants, looking at the effects of animal and plant foods on prostate cancer risk. The study found that men who ate the highest amount of dairy products had a 65 per cent higher risk of developing prostate cancer than those consuming the lowest amounts, whereas those who ate plant-based diets had a 36 per cent lower risk.[27] A correlation between an increased risk of prostate cancer and dairy consumption has also been found when comparing the incidence and mortality rates of prostate cancer in 42 countries alongside the dietary practices of the countries.[28] A review of three studies suggested that substituting one serving of dairy per day for nuts and legumes was associated with a 14 per cent lower risk of total mortality.[29]

Healthy plant-based sources of calcium include:

- Fortified plant milks
- Vegetables, such as kale, broccoli, bok choy and cabbage
- Legumes, such as beans and lentils
- Nuts, such as almonds, hazelnuts, walnuts, pistachios and Brazil nuts
- Seeds, such as chia and sesame (including tahini)
- Wholegrains, such as oats
- Dried fruits, such as figs, raisins, dried apricots and prunes

When it comes to calcium, certain foods, such as spinach, beet greens and Swiss chard, reduce the amount of calcium that can be absorbed by the body because they are high in oxalates. Cooking does however reduce the levels of these oxalates in the food, so it's not necessary to completely avoid these plants, especially as they are a great source of other nutrients, such as vitamin K and magnesium – they should just not be eaten too often and should preferably be cooked. Kale and broccoli, as well as being good sources of calcium (they actually have a higher calcium absorption rate than cow's milk),[30] are also low in oxalates. I like to add kale to a daily smoothie as it's an easy way of regularly getting calcium into my diet.

Vitamin D

Vitamin D helps the body to metabolise calcium, meaning that even if you are consuming the right amount of calcium, you won't absorb it properly if you are vitamin D deficient. Vitamin D is often called the sunshine vitamin, because sunlight is our main source. However, in many climates we are unable to rely on the sun to provide us with the vitamin D we need to be healthy during the winter months. That being said, I'm writing this on an overcast summer's day in the UK where it's more likely that I'll receive a vegan hamper from the NFU than my recommended amount of vitamin D from the sun. This is why it is recommended that everyone who lives in areas where there is limited access to sunlight should take a vitamin D3 supplement to make sure they are still getting the requisite amount, regardless of whether they eat a plant-based diet or not.

You can also get vitamin D from plant-based foods such as mushrooms that have been grown with UV light, as well as from fortified plant milks.

Omega-3

Much in the same way that calcium has become synonymous with cow's milk, omega-3 fatty acids have become exclusively linked with fish consumption, especially oily fish. Fat is an essential part of our diet that helps us to absorb vital nutrients, produces important hormones, provides energy and supports cell growth, among other things. However, there are different types of fat. Trans fat is a very harmful fat that can be found in heavily processed foods, such as fast food. Saturated fat is another harmful type of fat and is most commonly associated with meat, dairy and eggs but can also be found in high amounts in some plant-derived oils like coconut and palm. Consuming too much saturated fat has been linked to high cholesterol levels and an increased risk of heart disease.

However, unsaturated fats are an essential part of a healthy diet. Polyunsaturated fatty acids include an omega-3 (ALA) and an omega-6 fatty acid (LA) that are not made by the body so must be consumed through diet. The good news is that they are found in abundance in plant foods. Incorporating a tablespoon (or two) of ground flaxseed into your diet each day is a great way of getting the ALA your body needs and you can easily do this by adding it to a smoothie (along with the serving of kale I mentioned earlier). Personally, I like to get my daily amount of ground flaxseed by adding it to my morning oats.

However, it's true that the long-chain omega-3 fatty acids EPA and DHA that are also important for the body are virtually non-existent in plant foods. This is one reason why it's believed that it's necessary to eat fish or take supplements derived from fish. However, fish do not produce long-chain omega-3 fats themselves – the source of these fats in our diet is algae eaten by the fish. So this essentially means that we are filtering the nutrients through an animal unnecessarily when we could just consume it from the source instead by taking an algae oil supplement. Our bodies can convert ALA into both EPA and DHA, but the rates of conversion can vary, so an algae oil supplement is the best way of ensuring that you are consuming the recommended amount each day.

By getting long-chain omega-3 fats from algae oil supplements we are avoiding the saturated fat that is found in fish, not to mention the toxins and pollutants that they often contain, including mercury and micro-plastics. Ironically, the fish-farming industries often give algae oil to the fish to boost their long-chain omega-3 fats,[31] meaning we create the supplement and then give it to fish in aquatic factory farms that produce waste, pollution and greenhouse gas emissions, and that also cause huge amounts of suffering and disease that we then have to treat with antibiotics. All so we can then kill them and claim fish is a good source of omega-3 fats. It's cheaper, healthier, more sustainable, more ethical and reduces antibiotic resistance to just eat the supplement ourselves in the first place. Fish oil is already one of the most popular supplements, so for millions of people it's simply a case of changing the supplement to a different one.

The best sources of plant-based omega-3 fatty acids are:

- Ground flaxseed and flaxseed oil
- Chia seeds
- Hemp seeds
- Walnuts

B12

Vitamin B12 is often described as the Achilles heel of veganism, but that doesn't really hold up to scrutiny. It is made by microbes that are found in soil and are present in the digestive tracts of animals, including humans. However, our body is unable to absorb the B12 that is produced by the microbes in our colon, meaning that we have to get the vitamin from our diet.

B12 can be found in animal products when the animals have consumed food, faeces, soil or water that contains B12, or through ruminant animals who produce B12 in their digestive system when they consume the mineral cobalt. Because our plant foods are sanitised and washed, there's no

B12 left on plant foods, whereas in years gone by we would have consumed B12 from contaminated water and plant foods, as well as from eating animals.

Studies have shown that up to 40 per cent of people in Western countries have low or marginal B12 status, meaning that inadequate B12 intake is far from only being a vegan problem.[32] Moreover, similar to how farmed fish are supplemented with algae oil for long-chain omega-3 fats, factory-farmed animals are given fortified feed and supplemented with B12[33] because they're not getting B12 in the natural way either. Even grass-fed animals are often supplemented with B12 or cobalt – which is necessary for ruminant animals to produce B12 in their digestive system – because lots of soil is now cobalt-deficient. In essence, the majority of B12 in our diet is coming from a supplement one way or another. So we are faced with the choice of contributing to animal suffering, environmental degradation, an increased risk of infectious disease and antibiotic resistance to get B12, or we can take a supplement, which is more often than not the way the animals we consume get B12 in the first place. You can also get B12 from fortified plant foods such as cereals, plant milks and nutritional yeast, but it's still advisable to supplement B12 anyway.

Supplements

If I had a pound for every time someone told me that veganism is unhealthy because vegans take supplements, I would have enough to a buy a lifetime's supply of B12. However, the truth is that society has relied on supplementation and fortification for decades, and it's so normalised and widespread that we don't even recognise it. For example, outside of farmed fish being supplemented with long-chain omega-3 fatty acids and farmed terrestrial animals being supplemented with B12 or cobalt, the following supplements are widespread in our food chain:

- Cow's milk is often fortified with vitamin D, iodine and vitamin A
- Soils are often fortified with selenium and cobalt
- Cereal grain products such as bread and cereals are often fortified with nutrients such as folic acid, riboflavin, niacin, vitamin B6, pantothenic acid, iron, calcium and vitamin D
- Salt is often iodised, meaning it is mixed with iodine
- Flour is often fortified with iron
- Egg-laying hens are often given vitamin D and omega-3 supplements
- Animals are also often supplemented with selenium, zinc, iodine, vitamin E, phosphorus, copper

. . . And the list goes on. And this doesn't even take into account the 76 per cent of US adults[34] and 48 per cent of UK adults who take a supplement on a regular basis.[35] If it's unhealthy that vegans get some nutrients from a supplement or through fortified foods then it must be unhealthy that non-vegans do as well; so, by that logic, there should be no fortified foods for humans or fortified feeds and supplements for the animals we farm. While supplements shouldn't be taken as an excuse to not eat a healthy diet, complementing a diet that centres on whole-plant foods with a supplement is a great way of making sure you aren't missing out on anything your body needs. Plus, it also means that you are then able to take full advantage of the benefits of a wholefoods plant-based diet and the reductions in chronic disease it can bring.

I would recommend taking a supplement that is designed for vegans, meaning that it isn't just a general multivitamin that contains everything, which is unnecessary and can mean you are consuming more than the recommended daily dose of some nutrients. Most supplements for vegans will contain vitamin B12, vitamin D3, zinc, selenium, iron, vitamin K2 and iodine. Some will also contain long-chain omega-3 fats, but if not, I would include an algae oil supplement as well. It can also be useful to use a food-tracking app when you first go vegan, as that way you can monitor your calories and nutrients and make sure that you are meeting all of your recommended daily amounts.

On top of this, I would also recommend:

- Choose unsweetened and fortified plant milks – soya and oat are my favourite for their taste, nutritional profile and sustainability
- Take one or two tablespoons of ground flaxseed a day
- Avoid refined grains and opt for wholegrains, including wholewheat pasta, brown rice and brown bread
- Eat a Brazil nut daily for selenium
- Eat the rainbow – meaning eat a variety of different coloured fruits and vegetables (especially berries, dark leafy greens and cruciferous vegetables, such as cauliflower and kale)
- Limit processed foods and salt
- Drink plenty of water (about eight glasses a day)

AN OUNCE OF PREVENTION IS WORTH A POUND OF CURE

Eating a healthy plant-based diet also has the advantage of helping to prevent some of our most common chronic diseases, something that's predicted to become increasingly important in the near future. In the USA, 60 per cent of adults have a chronic disease and 40 per cent have two or more.[36] In the UK, it is predicted that by 2035, 67 per cent of over 65s will be living with two or more chronic diseases.[37] Consequently, understanding how our lifestyles impact our risks of developing chronic diseases and preventing them is becoming increasingly important. This is where the benefits of a wholefoods plant-based diet become particularly significant, as it's not only healthy from a nutritional perspective, it can even reduce the risk of many of our leading diseases and illnesses.

Although the prevalence of many diseases is increasing, wholefood plant-based diets have been shown to be low-risk interventions that are not only more cost effective than medications but also don't come with the side effects and negative consequences of pharmaceutical treatments. So how exactly does swapping from animal-based foods to plants help?

Heart Disease

Unfortunately, most of us will know someone who has had a heart attack or suffers from heart disease. It's an illness that we have become so used to that we almost passively accept it as an inevitable part of life. In fact, ischaemic heart disease is the number one killer globally, causing the deaths of about nine million people in 2019.[38] The condition arises when plaque, which is a build-up of fatty deposits, accumulates inside the coronary arteries, restricting the flow of blood to the heart and therefore oxygen around the body. The disease develops over a long period of time, with a progressive restriction of blood flow occurring. Angina, which is the sensation of pain and pressure around the heart, is a symptom of heart disease, as is breathlessness due to the decreased blood flow. A heart attack can then arise when the plaque inside the artery ruptures, leading to a clot forming that can cause a blockage and cut off the blood supply. In the USA, someone has a heart attack every 40 seconds.[39]

There are a range of risk factors associated with heart disease, including smoking and lack of exercise. However, according to one major analysis of 195 countries, diet is the largest risk factor when it comes to heart disease, with the findings showing that approximately 70 per cent of ischaemic heart disease deaths across the world could be prevented by people adopting healthier diets more focused on fruits, vegetables, nuts and wholegrains.[40]

Although we require some cholesterol to be healthy, our body produces all we need. When we consume diets high in saturated fat, cholesterol levels become raised beyond what is healthy, which in turn contributes to the hardening of arteries and the increased likelihood of a blood clot forming. A wholefoods plant-based diet does not contain any dietary cholesterol – a major study comparing the effects of plant-based diets and omnivorous diets on cholesterol levels found that plant-based diets are associated with decreased total cholesterol.[41] Importantly, it is also very low in saturated fat. Processed foods – whether vegan or containing animal products – can be high in trans fat, saturated fat and salt, so it is also important to avoid them whenever possible to reduce the risk of heart disease.

As we've seen, whole-plant foods are also high in fibre. In the case of heart disease, soluble fibre slows the absorption of cholesterol and reduces the amount produced by the liver. It can also reduce blood pressure and inflammation, two other important risk factors when it comes to heart disease.

Amazingly, a plant-based diet doesn't just help prevent heart disease but can even be of benefit to those who already have it. A plant-based intervention heart trial that was conducted in 2014 involved 198 people who had heart disease being put on a wholefoods plant-based diet. Of the 177 people who stuck with the diet, one of them had a stroke. However, of the 21 people who didn't stick with the diet, 13 of them suffered a cardiac event – meaning they either had a stroke, a heart attack or a bypass operation.[42]

Stroke

Almost 90 per cent of strokes are ischaemic,[43] meaning that they stem from blockages in the blood vessels leading to clots that deprive the brain of oxygen, which can cause leg and arm weakness, loss of speech, paralysis and death. While there has been less investigation into the role of plant-based diets and stroke risk, a wholefoods plant-based diet has been associated with a decreased likelihood, with one analysis finding that those who ate plant-based diets were associated with a 10 per cent lower risk of suffering a stroke.[44]

In 2019, a report was released that looked at 48,000 participants and determined that 'vegetarians' (in fact, a group that contained both vegans and vegetarians) had a 13 per cent lower rate of ischaemic heart disease but a 20 per cent higher risk of stroke, mainly because of higher rates of haemorrhagic strokes (which are caused when blood vessels burst).[45] This generated a huge amount of media attention. However, on closer evaluation, only 11 per cent of the vegetarian group were vegan, with the vegetarians in this grouping consuming 29 per cent more cheese than the meat eaters. Cheese is commonly high in saturated fat and salt, which are both major risk factors for high blood pressure and strokes. They were also consuming below the recommended daily amount of fibre,[46] which is important in the prevention of vascular disease. The meat eaters were also more likely to be taking medications to lower their cholesterol and blood pressure, which could have helped in reducing the risk of stroke. Plus, a 2016 report that combined the same data set and then also factored in another study as well, found no significantly higher risk of stroke mortality in vegetarians or vegans compared with meat eaters.[47]

One large review of studies into strokes discovered that those who had more than five servings of fruit and vegetables a day were associated with a 26 per cent lower than average risk of suffering a stroke.[48] A reason for this could be to do with antioxidants (compounds that can prevent the cells in our bodies from being damaged), which have been linked with lower stroke risk. Fruits and vegetables are among the best sources of antioxidants; in fact, on average, plants have 64 times more antioxidants than animal foods.[49] A study of Swedish women showed that those who ate the most antioxidant-rich foods were associated with the lowest risk of stroke.[50] Unfortunately, according to the CDC, only one in ten US citizens get even five servings of fruit and vegetables a day, let alone more than five.[51]

Dementia

The number of people living with dementia is increasing, and, as life expectancy goes up and we live longer lives, it is predicted to become even more common in the future. Alzheimer's disease is a progressive illness that causes memory loss, unstable moods, paranoia, confusion and death, and is the most prevalent form of dementia. While there is no proven way to reverse it, there are some preventative measures that can reduce the risk. According to the Alzheimer's Association, they include regular exercise, not smoking, limited alcohol intake, cognitively stimulating activities and a healthy diet.[52]

In a study of 6,000 Americans with an average age of 68, those eating a 'Mediterranean diet' – meaning a diet that includes fish but also more vegetables, wholegrains, beans, seeds, nuts and fruit and little red meat and dairy – were associated with a third lower risk of dementia. The lead author of the study stated, 'Eating a healthy plant-based diet is associated with better cognitive function and around 30 per cent to 35 per cent lower risk of cognitive impairment during aging.'[53]

In 2020, a large review study found that cholesterol is a risk factor for developing Alzheimer's disease.[54] This matches up with other studies that found that better heart health in midlife was associated with a lower risk of dementia.[55, 56, 57] Studies have also found that the brains of patients suffering from Alzheimer's disease have significant oxidative damage,[58] so eating antioxidant-rich plant foods could play a role in Alzheimer's-disease prevention. This was shown in one study that discovered that those participants who consumed the highest amount of plant-based flavonoids, a type of nutrient rich in antioxidants, were associated with a 40 per cent lower risk of developing dementia when compared to those with the lowest intake.[59]

The 2014 Dietary and Lifestyle Guidelines for the Prevention of Alzheimer's, which were developed as part of the International Conference on Nutrition and the Brain, also recommended that 'vegetables, legumes [beans, peas and lentils], fruits and whole grains should replace meats and dairy products as primary staples of the diet'.[60]

Diabetes

There are two main types of diabetes: type 1 and type 2. Ninety per cent of sufferers have type 2 diabetes, when the body becomes insulin resistant. This is primarily related to lifestyle choices, particularly diet.[61] Insulin is what normally allows blood sugar to enter muscle cells, where it can be stored and used for energy, but when fat builds up inside muscle and liver cells the insulin-signalling process is blocked, causing cells to reject the insulin. This leaves glucose stuck in the bloodstream, causing very high blood-sugar levels, which in turn leads to the pancreas creating more insulin that the body can't process.

Excess fat also leads to the death of beta cells, which are what produce insulin in the pancreas. The body stops producing beta cells around the time we turn twenty, which means that our ability to produce insulin decreases as these cells die, hence why type 2 diabetics can often need insulin injections.

Because insulin resistance causes blood sugar to spike, people often think that limiting carbohydrates, which provide the body with glucose, is the best way to treat type 2 diabetes. The problem with this approach is that it attempts to deal with a symptom of the problem not the problem itself.

While eliminating refined carbohydrates such as pastries and doughnuts is important, these foods are also high in saturated and trans fats and refined sugars, which are just as damaging. Complex carbohydrates, such as wholegrains, beans, vegetables, fruits and pulses, also create glucose in the body, but they don't have the same negative effects as refined carbohydrates – quite the opposite, in fact, as they are filled with fibre, antioxidants and other nutrients. Also, eating whole-plant foods means swapping saturated fat for mono-unsaturated and polyunsaturated fats, which have been shown to improve insulin resistance and insulin secretion.[62]

One major study found that those who ate a predominantly plant-based diet had a 23 per cent lower risk of type 2 diabetes. Another study found that those on a plant-based diet were associated with a 78 per cent lower risk of type 2 diabetes when compared to those who ate meat on a daily basis.[63] They were also associated with a 27 per cent lower risk than pescatarians, suggesting that to maximise the potential of diet we need to do more than just swap saturated fat for unsaturated fat – we also need to move to a diet of whole-plant foods.

As well as preventing type 2 diabetes, a plant-based diet can also help to reduce the impact of diabetes in people who already have it. In a groundbreaking study in Slovakia, 1,000 type 2 diabetics were placed on the Natural Food Interaction (NFI) protocol, an entirely plant-based diet. After 22 weeks, 84 per cent came off their medication because the disease had gone into remission.[64] The study was authored by the leading diabetes doctors and researchers in Slovakia and has been so influential that one of the major medical insurance companies in the country is now using the NFI protocol as a treatment for type 2 diabetes.[65]

Cancer

In 2015, the WHO's International Agency for Research on Cancer (IARC) released the findings of an analysis of more than 800 different studies on cancer in humans. They declared that processed meat is a class 1 carcinogen and that red meat is a class 2A carcinogen (class 1 being carcinogenic to humans and 2A probably being carcinogenic to humans).[66] While the conclusions were primarily based on the evidence of colorectal cancer, also referred to as bowel cancer, processed meat consumption was also associated with a higher risk of stomach cancer and red meat with a higher risk of pancreatic and prostate cancer.[67]

Researchers believe that the processing of the meat is one aspect of the problem, as smoking or curing, which involves adding nitrates, can potentially lead to the formation of cancer-causing chemicals. Haem iron was also cited as an increasing risk factor, as was the formation of cancer-causing chemicals that can be produced when meats are cooked at high temperatures, such as pan-frying, grilling and barbecuing.

In response to the research, a member of the Meat Advisory Board stated, 'What we do know is that avoiding red meat in the diet is not a protective strategy against cancer.'[68] They didn't, however, provide an analysis of more than 800 studies, including laboratory studies, to support that claim.

Colorectal cancer is the fourth leading cause of cancer-related deaths globally, with the number of deaths from the disease predicted to rise by 60 per cent by 2030.[69] Increasing rates of colorectal cancer correspond with a nation becoming more affluent and Westernised, suggesting that the lifestyle changes that accompany this transition are at least partly responsible.[70] One of the reasons suspected for this is the increased consumption of inflammatory diets. Pro-inflammatory foods include processed meat, red meat, organ meat, refined grains and sugary drinks. A study of more than 121,000 people showed that, even when adjusted for variables such as physical activity, men who ate the most inflammatory diets had a 44 per cent higher risk of developing colorectal cancer when compared to those eating the most anti-inflammatory diets. Women who ate the most inflammatory diets had a 22 per cent higher risk. Part of the problem could be that those consuming the most inflammatory diets also reported lower intakes of dietary fibre, dietary calcium and wholegrains.[71]

High levels of insulin like growth factor 1 (IGF-1) have also been linked to an increased risk of cancer. IGF-1 is a growth hormone that is produced by the liver and helps us to grow new tissue. However, when we have too much IGF-1, it can promote the growth and development of cancer. Eating animal products, including dairy, chicken and fish, increases the amount of IGF-1 in the body, while vegans have been shown to not only have reduced levels of IGF-1 but to also have higher levels of IGF-1 binding proteins, which are released by the liver to remove any excess IGF-1.[72]

The most comprehensive analysis that has been conducted exploring the relationship between IGF-1 and prostate cancer revealed that men who had the highest IGF-1 concentrations had a 29 per cent higher risk of prostate cancer compared to those with the lowest concentrations. And men with the highest IGF-1 binding proteins had a 19 per cent lower risk of prostate cancer compared to those who had the lowest.[73]

In the single largest study carried out investigating IGF-1 and breast cancer, the researchers found that those with the highest IGF-1 levels had a 37 per cent higher risk of breast cancer.[74]

Soy intake has also been associated with lower risk of cancer, with a study showing that women with the highest dietary soy intake were associated with a 12 per cent lower risk of breast cancer compared to those with the lowest intake.[75] For men, soy intake has been associated with a 29 per cent lower risk of prostate cancer.[76] And on the point of soy, there is a pervasive belief that soy intake has a feminising effect on men due to it containing phytoestrogens. However, phytoestrogens are plant hormones and don't have the same effect as oestrogen in the body. An analysis of 41 studies showed that intake of the plant does not affect testosterone levels in men,[77] and a narrative review of clinical evidence also showed that soy intake does not affect oestrogen levels in men, even at intake levels considerably higher than are typical for Asian males,[78] who have been shown to consume the most soy.

EMPOWERING OURSELVES THROUGH FOOD

When considering the mountain of evidence showing the dangers of animal consumption and the benefits of a plant-based diet, it's important to note that studies on human populations are far from perfect, as although they can identify correlations, they can't for the most part establish causations. This means that they don't definitively prove the associations they are showing. However, they can be used as a basis to establish links between hypotheses that can then be established more strongly with further observational studies, revealing patterns of associations. These associations can then be tested in clinical trials and intervention studies.

At this point, however, there is incontrovertible evidence linking the consumption of animal products with many of our leading chronic diseases and killers. While it's really important to note that diet and lifestyle should complement medical treatments and not be used to replace the advice of medical practitioners, it's also empowering to know that we can positively influence our health through our everyday choices.

We absolutely should be knowledgeable about where we are getting our nutrients from and make sure we are confident that we are obtaining everything we need to be healthy. It is beyond doubt that the benefits of a wholefoods plant-based diet, when combined with other lifestyle factors such as exercise, have the potential to reduce our risk of developing some of the most debilitating and severe chronic diseases that affect us.

The researchers behind the EAT-*Lancet* planetary health diet that I referenced earlier predict that switching to a more plant-based diet, which in Western countries, according to their analysis, would mean around an 80 per cent reduction in red meat, a six-fold increase of beans and lentil consumption, a fifteen-fold increase of nuts and seeds consumption, and an increase in the consumption of wholegrains, fruits and vegetables, could save at least 11 million people a year from deaths caused by eating unhealthy foods.[79, 80] Another study, this time by researchers at the University of Oxford, predicted that a global switch to more plant-based diets could save 8.1 million people from dying prematurely before the age of 75 by 2050.[81]

And it's not just about fewer deaths – switching to veganism has the potential to create a better quality of life, allowing people to reduce their reliance on certain medications and alleviate the symptoms caused by many of these diseases. Kaiser Permanente, one of the largest healthcare providers in the USA, has even told physicians to promote plant-based diets to their patients because it is a low-risk intervention that is cost effective and can treat multiple chronic illnesses at the same time.[82] And one of the most exciting aspects of a wholefoods plant-based diet is that it isn't one diet that can reduce heart-disease risk, another that can reduce diabetes risk and another that can reduce colorectal-cancer risk – it's the same diet.

So, although we can't ever eliminate the risk of these chronic diseases, it's at least rewarding to know that more wholegrains, legumes, beans, nuts, seeds, fruits and vegetables can certainly help. Ultimately, veganism is not just the best way to reduce animal suffering, it can also help stop us developing many of the most prevalent chronic diseases, meaning we live longer and healthier lives, which is something we can all surely aspire to.

PART THREE

BREAKING DOWN THE BARRIERS

7.

HOW PSYCHOLOGICAL BARRIERS INFLUENCE US

When I was a child, one of my favourite films was *Chicken Run*, an animation about a group of chickens living on an egg farm who are desperate to escape as the farmers are going to kill them and put them in a pie. I would root for these poor animals and hope they managed to evade the evil farmers, while simultaneously hoping that I was going to have chicken nuggets for dinner.

It is ironic that so many films and TV shows for kids feature the animals that we farm and kill by the billions. *Peppa Pig* is a well-known example, as is *Shaun the Sheep*, both beloved by children. Parents would be understandably outraged if Peppa was forced into a gas chamber in one episode or Shaun had his throat cut. And yet most parents are paying for those things to happen to real animals and feeding them to their children, who probably aren't even aware that the sausages they had for dinner came from a pig.

As children, our views of animals are very different to those we have as we grow older. Children don't evaluate the lives of animals based on what they do for us or what we can take from them; instead, they value them simply because of their existence.[1] A young child doesn't think it's wrong to hurt a dog because we culturally keep dogs as pets, but as they grow older that's what we teach them to believe. Likewise, in some areas of the world, children are taught that it's wrong to kill a cow. Essentially, as we grow older, we are taught that some animals have little intrinsic value beyond what they can provide for us. This is so heavily shaped by culture and historical precedence, as opposed to any objective and indisputable facts, that these taught values require us to create rationalisations and defences to justify what we do to certain animals.

A piglet makes us smile in the same way as a puppy; a little lamb is as cute as a kitten. We even take our children to petting zoos and open farms so that they can bottle-feed baby animals because it makes them, and us, happy. However, the child doesn't know, and the parent might not realise, that the child is fattening up the animal to be slaughtered.

Not long before I became vegan, I went to a small farm that was open to the public. I remember standing with one of the young farmers next to a pig pen, throwing food into it. The farmer told me that he was really happy because he had passed his driving test and was now able to drive the pigs to the slaughterhouse himself. I suddenly realised that I was fattening up the pigs for slaughter, and I was shocked by the farmer's excitement at being able to drive them to their death in the coming weeks. The happiness these pigs were providing me turned to guilt. These pigs thought they were being cared for and the smiles and laughter of those who came to visit them most likely assured them that they were safe. But they weren't. Far from it.

It would be heartbreaking for most children if they were told that the little lamb they were feeding was in a matter of months going to be slaughtered. And imagine if the farmer tried to slaughter the animal right there in front of everyone – the child would be traumatised, but, then again, so would most of us. If we saw a chick being thrown into a macerator, we would be devastated. If we saw a piglet being mutilated, we would be deeply upset. If a farmer attempted to kill an animal in front of us, many of us would try to stop them. Yet these things happen every day, and we pay for them to happen. We don't think about it – we choose not to think about it – because it is out of sight and out of mind. We form deep psychological defence mechanisms as we grow older, and these industries are able to make great profits doing things we would try to stop if they were happening in our presence.

To illustrate my point, let's say the next time you are out walking, you see someone attacking a dog with the intention of killing them. What do you do? Do you try to intervene? Do you call the police? Do you try to save the dog's life? What if instead of a dog the animal being attacked and killed in front of you was a pig – do you still try to save their life? Now let's say you are walking home and a pig is being attacked and killed, except it's not happening in front of you but is instead taking place in a room in a building we call a slaughterhouse – does that remove the need for you to intervene? Is unnecessarily killing a pig always wrong or just when it's happening right in front of you?

ACKNOWLEDGING THE INDIVIDUAL

One of the most significant demonstrations of this attitude in practice is how we react when animals escape slaughter. In 2019, a cow affectionately named Daisy by people online escaped from a slaughterhouse in Carlisle, England. Daisy ran into a nearby cul-de-sac and prompted a huge outcry from people wishing for her to be rescued, even though she was running away from a fate that is determined by the actions of many of these people, most of whom would happily have eaten her had she not escaped. The police ended up shooting Daisy and killing her, leading to public condemnation.[2]

This story reveals so much about how we view animals and their slaughter. The fact that we yearn for escaped animals to live speaks volumes about how we value their lives once they become separated from the anonymous herd. We then acknowledge that they are individuals with their own personalities and a clear desire to live. We recognise that there is something they are trying to escape from, that they are fearful and in a situation they do not want to be in, which is so troubling that they would rather take the risk of running into the unknown than allow what is happening to them to continue. In essence, we view these animals as underdogs, heroes overcoming adversity, and yet the adversity they are trying to overcome is us. They're only there because of the choices that we make. These animals are not simply escaping the slaughterhouse or trying to evade the police. They are running from us, the people who have decided their fate long before they were born. It may be the slaughterer's knife or a police officer's bullet that physically kills the animals, but their deaths are on all our hands.

This is another reason why animals who escape slaughter make such an impact on us – they defy the perceptions that we have of them. They display sentience and emotion and expose our preconception that they are unintelligent, biological machines who have no idea what's happening to them and don't really care as false. The problem is we then view that one animal as being special; we determine that they deserve life because they're not like all the other animals. However, there is no reason why that animal is more deserving of life; it's just that our perception of them has changed.

Another revealing aspect of stories like this one is the idea that animals must fight for their freedom and earn the right to live. However, it shouldn't be the case that just because others are unable to make a break for freedom their deaths become more justifiable as a result. We don't apply this standard to other situations of animal suffering, such as dogs being farmed in South East Asia. We would never say that only the ones who are able to escape shouldn't be killed.

These examples reveal one of the main ways in which we psychologically excuse what we do to animals. Just as the dog and pig thought experiment showed us we would feel responsible for an animal being hurt or killed in front of us, seeing animals escape and become publicly visible creates a similar sense of culpability. On some level, whether consciously for some or unconsciously for others, we understand our role in what is happening and feel guilty as a result. Basically, the animal's suffering is no longer out of sight and out of mind, as it is normally. When we are not directly confronted with what happens to millions of animals every day, we can psychologically distance ourselves from it.

The aphorism 'if slaughterhouses had glass walls, we'd all be vegetarian' expresses a significant idea. We are so detached from what happens that we never think about it. We buy a steak in a supermarket but never stop to consider the cow who has been killed. We buy a bacon sandwich but never think about the pig in the gas chamber. We are removed from the process and therefore able to absolve ourselves of any responsibility – ignorance, after all, is bliss.

This is exactly how the animal-product industries want us to feel and why they are shrouded in secrecy. There are even laws in the USA, Australia and Canada known as 'ag-gag laws', which make it illegal to film farms and slaughterhouses. If an investigator or journalist in Iowa, for example, went onto a farm and secretly filmed an animal being abused in an illegal way, they could be jailed for two years,[3] which is the same sentence that the person caught abusing the animal could receive.[4]

In the UK in late 2019, a farm part owned by the deputy president of the NFU at that time was exposed for illegal treatment of animals, including beatings and sexual abuse.[5] In response, a spokesperson for the farm stated, 'Trespassers entered our farm unlawfully and secretly filmed many hours of footage . . . We regard this as a gross breach of privacy . . . and absolutely condemn it.'[6] There is such reluctance to acknowledge what happens in farms and slaughterhouses that even though the investigation was not illegal and exposed great wrongdoing, the industry was keener to condemn the investigation than what had been exposed.

These kinds of responses are of course attempts to deflect blame from what is happening to the animals and undermine the investigations but I also think there is something less obvious going on as well, something that in turn points to a wider problem related to farming and indeed animal-product consumption more generally.

REVEALING OUR DISSONANCE: FROM UFOS TO FIREFIGHTERS

Cognitive dissonance is a psychological concept that was identified by Leon Festinger in the 1950s. It is described as the psychological stress that occurs when a person's beliefs, values or ideas contradict or go against an action or behaviour that they are engaged in. The concept came from a study of a cult in Chicago that believed a UFO was going to rescue them from a cataclysmic event due to cause huge destruction across the world. When the event didn't happen, and a UFO didn't come to save them, the followers of the cult convinced themselves that it was going to happen a few days later. When the next predicted day came and went, the followers were forced to confront the dissonance that they were experiencing. Many members of the group returned home and recognised the falsity of what they had believed; however, others declared that their faith had saved the world from the event – the aliens were no longer coming to rescue them because they had stopped the disaster from taking place.

Dissonance becomes most evident when it threatens our belief that we are kind, ethical and competent. And as seen in this case study, when someone is confronted with dissonance, they have two choices: they can either change their behaviour or attempt to justify it. While this was a blatant form of cognitive dissonance in action, there are more subtle and societally accepted instances. For example, our desire for cheap clothes contradicts our shared value of being against human exploitation and, in the case of what we do to animals, our desire to eat animal products contradicts our being against animal cruelty.

When farmers' malpractices are exposed, this undermines their beliefs that they are kind and ethical and they must either accept the truth or justify why they are not in the wrong, such as claiming that those responsible for the investigation are acting illegally. As consumers, our cognitive dissonance means we often believe these are just bad apples, that they don't represent the industry as a whole and don't reveal a systemic problem. And yet by this point there have surely been enough bad apples to suggest that the whole tree is rotten.

Another good example of the cognitive dissonance of consumers is demonstrated by the story of a man in Florida who pleaded guilty to nine animal-cruelty charges for killing nine ducklings by running them over with a lawnmower and macerating them. He was sentenced to a year in jail, with three years of probation, and was ordered to have a mental-health evaluation.[7] However, is it not jarring that macerating nine ducklings constitutes nine separate charges of animal cruelty but killing 7 billion male chicks every single year as soon as they are born, often by macerating them in grinders, is not only viewed as acceptable but is often defended by people who claim that it is those who do not believe in killing male chicks who are extreme? How can it be wrong to kill nine ducklings but not billions of male chicks, especially considering both acts are ultimately needless?

This example demonstrates an obvious contradiction, which speaks to the wider issue of our cognitive dissonance in relation to animal product consumption. The reality is that if we took the legally sanctioned practices from the animal farming industries and then applied them to other situations, we would think those practices horrendous. For example, if dog owners were cutting off their pets' tails and chopping their teeth out, we would condemn that as being horrific animal abuse. But we do it to pigs and call it high welfare. If someone was killing puppies by thumping their heads against a wall or dislocating their necks, we would call that evil, yet that happens to animals such as piglets and chickens and we call it humane. But the experience is the same for the individual animal, regardless of what species they are.

In another example, firefighters in the UK rescued eighteen piglets and two breeding sows from a farm barn that had caught fire. The farmer who owned the pigs later had them slaughtered and turned into sausages, which she then gave to the firefighters as a thank you for rescuing them.[8] The firefighters said, 'We can tell no porkies, the sausages were fantastic.'

While the fact that the firefighters rescued the pigs in the first place shows that they have compassion and empathy for animals, if they had not done so, it would have been considered incredibly immoral. Vegans were upset that the firefighters ate the pigs, but there would have been condemnation from non-vegans and vegans alike if the firefighters had actively chosen to let the pigs burn. However, the suffering of the animals in a barn fire and the suffering in a slaughterhouse are equally as unwanted and just as likely to cause pain. So, why do we consider it right to save animals from unnecessary suffering in one situation but not in another, when they would wish to be saved in either case?

RE-EVALUATING OUR UNDERSTANDING OF ANIMALS

Another major way in which we devalue the intelligence of farmed animals, and thereby psychologically justify our treatment of them, is by viewing them as all being the same. One of the reasons for this is that we have bred them to be genetically similar, which further plays into the idea that they are just a collective mass that lack any significant or meaningful individuality. When we remove characteristics or traits that would make it easier to see them as individuals, we instead view them as a mass of interchangeable 'things'. Fish are of course the ultimate abstraction – thousands of species all categorised as if they are merely one. We remove all individualism from them, and, even with all the scientific evidence that supports the fact they feel pain,[9] we still treat them as if they are nothing more than inanimate ocean objects.

Perpetuating the idea that animals aren't individuals or worthy of any regard allows us to characterise them in a way that suits our desire to eat them. This is why we refer to pigs as being dirty and chickens as being stupid. These characterisations further reinforce the idea that non-human animals are not morally relevant and it is therefore acceptable to cause them harm, because they are cognitively inferior.

Interestingly, in one study, undergraduate students were asked to fill out a survey ranking the traits of chickens, such as their intelligence, their capacity to feel and their individual personalities. Afterwards, the students had a practical class with live chickens where they used positive reinforcement to teach the chickens tricks. They were then asked to do the same survey again and the students rated the intelligence and presence of individual personalities in chickens more highly this time around. In their written feedback, students included statements like, 'Interesting that chickens are a lot smarter than I originally thought.'[10]

The fact that the students ranked the chickens low to begin with speaks volumes about our initial perception of these animals. We essentially think of them as being dissimilar to us and even accuse people who say that animals have emotions of anthropomorphising them, or criticise those who say that animals value their lives, mourn being separated from their babies or don't want to die, as if it were only humans who can experience emotions and desire. The obvious reality is that if we acknowledged that animals are capable of these emotions and feelings, we would struggle to diminish their worth to the point whereby doing everything that we do to them becomes morally acceptable.

A report that the UK was considering banning the importation of foie gras prompted the director of the industry's association, the Comité Interprofessionnel des Palmipèdes à Foie Gras, to state that there is a 'problem of judgements based on anthropomorphic perceptions that the animal used in the production is suffering . . . People have to stop imagining a tube being inserted in their own throat, because a duck and goose's throat is nothing like yours.'[11] It's no wonder this position is taken by the industry, as they confine animals in cages, force feed them twice a day so that their livers grow to seven to ten times their normal size[12] and then cut their throats. Not to mention that studies have shown that force-fed birds have mortality rates ten to twenty times higher than non-force-fed birds.[13] So it's hardly surprising that the industry feels the need to discredit the suffering of these animals, because if they viewed what they were doing objectively, they would either have to leave the industry and their livelihoods or spend every day consciously causing horrendous, needless suffering. Ignorance is bliss, even when it's wilful.

However, sometimes farmers react differently. One sheep farmer who had been in the animal farming industry for 47 years decided he couldn't live with taking his animals to slaughterhouses any more and drove his lambs to an animal sanctuary instead. He also stopped eating meat at the same time and switched to farming vegetables, allowing the cattle he already had to live out the rest of their lives with him on the farm.[14] In another example, a dairy farmer interviewed on a BBC programme called *The Dark Side of Dairy* broke down when asked about the process of separating calves from their mothers, saying that there were mother cows who would 'bawl for days'.[15] No doubt many other dairy farmers would accuse him of anthropomorphising cows.

SOMEONE NOT SOMETHING

There are a number of further ways in which we attempt to distance ourselves from what happens to animals and one of those is through our use of language. A common term used to describe animals who we farm is 'livestock'. By referring to them as livestock we create a distinction between farm animals and the others that exist in the world. It essentially 'otherises' the animals we exploit and places them in a different classification, which in turn further perpetuates the idea that it is acceptable to use and kill them. The word livestock further commodifies these animals, as we literally classify them as being 'stock' – as for a shelf, a product that we can trade and profit from. But, of course, there's no difference between the animals we call livestock and the animals we don't except our perception of them. 'Livestock' only comes as a plural – it forces us to see the animals as a group rather than identifying with an individual. To see them as being a something rather than a someone. You might have also noticed that I very deliberately refer to animals as 'he', 'she', 'they' or 'who' rather than 'it' or 'that'. Animals are not inanimate objects; they are living beings, and the language we use to describe them is important.

This concept of categorising animals allows our values to fluctuate, especially considering that the number of animals we deem to be 'food' is an incredibly small fraction of all the edible animals that exist. A fascinating example of this was the scandal in Europe in 2013 when many beef products, such as burgers and lasagnes, were found to contain horse meat. People in the UK were outraged that they were consuming horses and not cattle, although morally there's no difference. Horse meat is widely consumed across many areas of Europe, tastes similar to cattle flesh and even has twice as much iron as steak from a cow.[16] And the UK is one of the biggest horse-racing nations in the world, with many horses dying on the track each year, often with a black curtain pulled around them so that they can be shot out of sight. Hundreds of racehorses are slaughtered[17] and often exported to places in Europe where they will be eaten.[18] So, by British standards, it's acceptable to shoot a horse on a racetrack, it's even acceptable to kill them in a slaughterhouse, but eating them is immoral and scandalous.

The species of animals we consider to be 'food animals' have changed over time. Up until the 1930s, people in the UK did eat horse meat.[19] In the 1950s, whale meat was available to buy in the UK and was called 'whacon', which the UK government recommended for its high nutritional value.[20] After the Second World War, whale meat was even 'off ration', meaning it could be distributed without restriction. Today, most British people would baulk at the idea of eating horse or whale flesh.

An argument that is often used to justify eating the animals we do is that we have eaten them for millennia. But the same is also true of dog meat, with dogs being consumed in Germany[21] in the early twentieth century, and they are still consumed in rural areas of Switzerland.[22] Incidentally, dog meat is high in protein and iron (it too can contain more than beef), an argument that is often used to justify consuming animal flesh – for its 'nutritional value'. I can't imagine that dog lovers across the UK would be happy with someone cutting a dog's throat because their flesh is a good source of iron and protein, yet self-professed animal lovers can pay for a cow's throat to be cut and defend that action with the same logic.

The problem is that once an animal is classified as being 'food', the way we think about that animal's attributes changes. This is why the fact that cattle flesh is high in protein is used as a justification for what we do to them, yet the fact that dogs, cats, whales and many other edible animals are also high in protein doesn't then make us feel differently about consuming them. Imagine how people would react if someone bred dogs into existence, gave them six months of life and then cut their throats with the justification: 'I gave them a good life, I cut their throat humanely, I like how they taste and they're a good source of essential nutrients, such as protein and zinc. Besides, people have been eating dogs for thousands of years, and it's not right for you to force your views on me.' It's interesting that millions of people sign petitions condemning dog-meat consumption in Asia, but if a vegan questions their consumption of other animals, the vegan is forcing their views on them.

PROCESSING FACT FROM FICTION

I t's not just the word livestock that distances us from what is happening to animals. The animal-agriculture industries constantly use euphemisms to try to mask what is really happening. For example, I was having a conversation with a farmer who told me that they don't use the word slaughter any more and instead say that the animals are 'harvested' and then 'processed'. In fact, in 2019, at the New South Wales annual farming conference, farmers voted for the word 'slaughter' to be completely removed from their promotional material and replaced with the word 'processed', as they believed that the former was too emotive and undermined people's trust in animal farming. One animal farmer in attendance said, 'The word slaughter is not appropriate for our industry.'[23]

This hypocrisy is also demonstrated by what many animal products are called, with some named in such a way that we are disconnected from the reality of who we are eating. Even though the origins of many of these words can be traced back hundreds of years, it's interesting to note that referring to animal flesh as meat, pig flesh as pork, cattle flesh as beef and baby cow flesh as veal, among others, further detaches us from having to think about the animals whose bodies we are purchasing and consuming.

Imagine if supermarkets called their meat sections 'dead animal' aisles. Or if instead of bacon we bought 'sliced pig flesh' and on the packaging it explained the process of how they were gassed to death. By turning animals into objects, classifying them differently and using different words to describe them when they are living and when they are dead, it helps us to avoid the discomfort of thinking of them in gas chambers or hung up on the kill line about to have their throats cut.

ACKNOWLEDGING OUR IMPERFECTIONS

But, of course, there's more to the psychology of animal product consumption than our attempt to 'otherise' animals and diminish their experiences. As humans, we are capable of truly remarkable things; however, despite our intelligence, we are susceptible to cognitive biases and imperfections and vulnerabilities in our thinking that can get in the way of rational or objective decision-making. One of the most prevalent is confirmation bias, where our brains view information that agrees with our preconceptions as being more important than information that contradicts them. The information we are first taught is fundamental to how we perceive the world as we develop and is very difficult to dislodge, even when there is good evidence that it is wrong. Confirmation bias also means that we are more likely to look for information and read articles or resources that agree with our pre-existing beliefs or opinions, which is why a negative article about veganism can go viral and every vegan hears about it from their meat-eating friends but a piece of research supporting veganism doesn't get the same kind of reaction.

There's also false-consensus bias, whereby we believe that something must be acceptable because the majority of people do it. However, there have been many examples throughout history where something was socially accepted and the majority of people were active participants at that time but the practice was later rejected. It's understandable that we find comfort in being a part of the crowd. First, because it makes us feel like we are sharing the burden of responsibility, and any moral issues are diffused as a result of the action being collective rather than individualistic. In essence, we are relinquishing part of our agency in return for the peace of mind that comes with surrendering part of our responsibility. And second, the perceived comfort of being a part of the collective also comes from a more deeply entrenched fear of being ostracised.

We have always been social animals, reliant on the safety of being part of the tribe or community. Indeed, our very survival has, throughout most of our history, been dependent on being part of a collective. So when we do something that goes against the group and defies the values of the majority, we are in effect ostracising ourselves from the community. Psychologically speaking, this is a terrifying prospect, as we view ostracisation as not only being negative but potentially catastrophic. This is why one of the most important aspects of the growth and normalisation of veganism is that as more people go vegan, it becomes viewed as less of a 'fringe' belief, and the fear of being detached from the collective will be removed.

To illustrate this point, one of the earliest pieces of research on social conformity, conducted in the 1950s, was the Asch Experiment, in which groups of up to eight participants were shown a card with a line on it. This was then followed by another card that had three lines labelled A, B and C. The participants then had to state out loud which of the three lines was the same as the one on the original card. To begin with, everyone in the group selected the correct lines; however, only one member of the group was actually being studied – the other members were all working with the researchers. As the test progressed, those who were involved in the research began to select the wrong answer on purpose, with 12 of the total 18 questions being answered incorrectly. The person who was being studied was positioned so that they would always either answer last or second to last, meaning they had plenty of time to think about the correct line but could also potentially be impacted by the answers of the others in the room. The research found that only 24 per cent of participants didn't conform on any question, with 75 per cent conforming at least once and 5 per cent conforming on every single question. In the control group, where there was no external pressure, only one subject gave a wrong answer.[24]

As humans we also have a proclivity for maintaining the status quo, which is another cognitive bias that can make us apprehensive of change and lead to us making decisions that ensure things stay mostly the same. We are also habitual in our decision-making. This makes the prospect of changing how we eat and live challenging, because it requires us to create new habits, which can be daunting. This is why we often find it easier to bury our heads in the sand, sometimes referred to as 'the ostrich effect' – a cognitive bias that can cause us to avoid things that we perceive as being unpleasant or challenging.

A good example of this is that many people will decline to watch footage from a slaughterhouse, saying something like, 'I don't want to watch that. It will put me off my food.' This is an interesting statement; after all, if we can't watch it with our own eyes, why is it acceptable for us to pay for it to happen? The reluctance to watch unpleasant footage surely defies the idea that what happens to animals is humane. If it were, surely it wouldn't be a problem for us to watch it in the first place.

We often spare little time to think of the reasons why we do what we do. We simply do it because we always have, those around us are doing it and we like it. But if we had to come face to face with the animals who were suffering on our behalf and press the button that lowered them into the gas chamber or pull the blade across their throat, perhaps we would think more about the consequences of our actions.

As consumers, we like to believe that we are exercising our free will and making our own personal choices when we buy the foods that we do. But does buying products that increase suffering really align with how we want the world to look? If our desire is for animals not to suffer, if we would actively intervene if a dog or a pig was being killed in front of us, if we root for an animal when they escape slaughter, if we would save a piglet from a burning fire, if we say we are against animal cruelty, then by buying animal products we are not living by our own preferences or in alignment with our values. We are doing the opposite. Our will is being manipulated to make us go against our intrinsic values. So perhaps it's time for us to turn our dissonance into harmony; something that is only possible once we recognise how our decision-making is being influenced.

HINDSIGHT IS GOOD, FORESIGHT IS BETTER

By acknowledging and understanding the psychological barriers that impact the choices we make, we can then critically reflect on our motivations for doing what we do. Without realising it, the consumption of animal products, which appears to be a surface-level and instinctual decision, is actually determined by an extensive amount of social and psychological rationales. It is also a decision that we spare very little time actively thinking about, even though it has such a huge impact.

I know from conversations I have had with other vegans that the biggest regret many of us feel is that we didn't go vegan sooner. I've seen people become really upset as they've admitted that they knew all the reasons they should become vegan but didn't because they kept trying to find a reason not to or expressed remorse that they were vegetarian for years but didn't make that extra step because they 'loved cheese too much'. Although hindsight makes it easy to regret such things, the reality is that making the change means confronting the barriers that can make it seem more comfortable and convenient to simply not worry about the issue of animal exploitation. However, we do have the foresight to know what will happen if we continue to exploit animals. This is why it is important to be conscious consumers, as our decision to perpetuate animal exploitation relies on us either being unconscious in our decision-making or wilfully ignoring the facts. But although the initial change can seem daunting, uncomfortable and inconvenient, the consequences of refusing to reflect on our actions and change accordingly will inevitably be much worse.

8.

WE HAVE NOTHING TO FEAR FROM INSTITUTIONAL AND MEDIA BIAS

The media holds a huge amount of influence over us, shaping our perceptions of certain topics by setting the agenda, deciding what is newsworthy and influencing how we feel through the way stories are framed. In essence, bias from the media can create bias in society as well. This is important, as it's highly likely that you have seen reports about veganism in the news with headlines such as 'Militant Veganism Is Out of Control'[1] or 'Farmers Sent Death Threats by Vegan Activists'.[2]

A good case in point occurred back in early 2018 when the BBC ran a piece about a farmer called Alison Waugh who said that she had received death threats and been sent notes from animal rights activists telling her and her family to 'go die'.[3] This caused a huge outcry, with national press coverage declaring that farmers were living in fear of vegans. I was subsequently invited onto the BBC to have a debate on live television with a dairy farmer about what they referred to as militant veganism and animal rights.

Waugh later stated that she had 'not had people making specific death threats towards me'.[4] Although this entirely contradicted her original statement, it had no effect on diminishing the narrative of frightened farmers living in fear of militant vegans who were sending death threats, nor did the BBC amend their original piece to reflect Waugh's retraction. Furthermore, every time I have been invited to discuss the narrative of frightened farmers and militant vegans in the media, I have always raised the point that I have received threats from farmers, butchers and meat eaters, yet the reaction to the threats I've received has never seemed as impassioned as the reaction that farmers get. Interestingly, I am always asked, 'Do you denounce vegans sending death threats?' I think my interviewers secretly hope that I will say no. However, I bet they've never been asked to denounce meat eaters sending death threats to vegans.

For example, Jude Capper, the founder of the pro-dairy campaign FebruDairy, set up to counteract Veganuary, was also involved in the BBC debate and was actively perpetuating the vegans-sending-farmers-death-threats narrative. However, during this time, Jude also liked a tweet talking about shooting vegans that said, 'Just load both barrels . . . but if you do shoot any vegans remember to dispose of their bodies in an environmentally friendly manner.'[5] Of course, it's unlikely there was any real intention behind the tweets but just imagine what the response would have been if the co-founders of Veganuary had liked a jokey tweet about shooting farmers.

It is clear, then, that the media latched onto this particular story not because they were outraged about the threats per se – unfortunately, most outspoken people on social media have received threats in one form or another – but because it played into a deeper narrative: the portrayal of veganism and animal rights as being militant, problematic and dangerous, something that exists outside of normalised society and poses a direct threat to its citizens and traditions. It's one of the oldest tricks in the book: the *ad hominem* attack of those who want to disrupt the status quo. Personal attacks are an effective way of avoiding debating the actual issues – if you can't argue against the message, you attack the messenger to try to muddy their public image and portray them in a way that puts people off.

MERCHANTS OF DOUBT

A great example of just this sort of media bias was seen in the *Daily Express* in 2018, which ran with the headline, 'Vegan Activists Want Farmers' Children HURT as Veggie Politics Get VERY DARK';[6] however, the article included no evidence to support that claim, and further assertions that 'vegans' strong viewpoints have led many to advocate the murder, rape and torture of farmers and their families' were provided with no supporting evidence either. Regardless of how baseless the claims were, this kind of messaging further reinforces the notion that outspoken vegans are a threat and something to be wary of.

The media also often falsely claims that young women, the demographic currently most likely to go vegan, are making the change due to having orthorexia and other eating disorders that they want to disguise. This is further combined with reports about veganism being unhealthy, with the death of a climber on Everest becoming a global news story because she was vegan,[7] even though many non-vegans have died climbing Everest and vegans have also climbed Everest and survived. More insidiously, veganism has been blamed for parents killing their children, with a story in 2007 exclaiming 'vegan diet kills baby',[8] even though the prosecutors in the case stated that, 'The child died because he was not fed. The vegan diet is fine.'[9] The narrative became that the baby died because the parents were vegan, not because they starved the baby by not feeding him.

Reports like this show a clear and emphatic bias. When babies of non-vegan parents die from malnourishment and starvation, they are never described as 'meat-eating killers', nor is the fact that the parents eat meat, dairy and eggs described as a reason for the baby dying. In 2020, I came across an article with the headline, 'Screaming Baby Starved to Death Surrounded by Curdled Milk As Mother Did Nothing.'[10] Throughout the article, there was no mention that the baby's mother ate animal products, but there is no doubt that the article would have read very differently if the baby had been surrounded by curdled soy milk.

These kinds of stories have a huge influence on people's perception of vegans, to the point where feeding certified class-one carcinogens, such as bacon, to children is seen as being an example of normal parenting but a plant-based diet is seen as child abuse. In 2019, a report came out attempting to discredit the WHO's advice to reduce processed and red-meat consumption on the grounds of an increased risk of cancer and heart disease.[11] The report was heavily criticised by public health researchers, including the American Heart Association,[12] the American Cancer Society[13] and the Harvard T.H. Chan School of Public Health.[14] It was also conducted by a research group that received funding from AgriLife, an organisation that works with the Texas Beef Checkoff and includes a beef cattle teaching programme, educational workshops for cattle ranchers and promotion of Texas beef to consumers, further undermining its impartiality.

However, this wasn't enough to stop Phillip Schofield, one of the most popular presenters on British television, defiantly declaring on a live broadcast to millions of people that 'bacon is back on the menu' and 'the bottom line is . . . when you read this stuff [the studies linking processed and red meat to cancer and heart disease], just think "Ah, I can't be bothered." Don't take any notice of them because they all change it.'[15] This statement was delivered to the British public as heart disease continues to be the number one killer of people worldwide[16] and colon cancer continues to be the second most deadly cancer in the UK,[17] with only lung cancer killing more people each year. Unfortunately, examples like this don't just turn people away from veganism, they potentially compromise people's health and lives.

I came face to face with Phillip Schofield when I appeared on *This Morning* in late 2018 to discuss 'militant' veganism with him, his co-host Rochelle Humes and the journalist Julie Bindel, who was appearing as a guest alongside me, in a segment very subtly called 'Are Militant Vegans Going Too Far?'[18] Even though I had expected that I would be asked to denounce death threats, the lengths that the show went to try to get me to say something that would insinuate that I have nefarious intentions was surprising, and it wasn't until after the interview that I realised how significantly Phillip had tried to goad me into a reaction:

Phillip: Are you militant?

Me: Militant is an interesting word. I stand up for what I believe in and I speak it and I preach it, and I do it hopefully in a way that I believe to be effective.

Phillip: How far will you go?

Me: How far will I go? I mean, that sounds like a loaded question.

Phillip: Well, it is a loaded question . . .

Me: Exactly.

Phillip: Because obviously we're talking, we're going to talk about the, the, the militant vegans . . .

Me: Yeah.

Phillip: And so when I use that word, you say you don't really like it but who will take it to the extreme? Who will be violent? Who will be offensive? Who will be frankly quite frightening?

Me: Right. So violence of course is never on the table. We don't condone violence in any way, shape or form. Offence is a very unique thing – it's very subjective. I'm personally offended by people who exploit animals; however, my offence about it isn't necessarily a good enough justification for them just to stop. So, we have to not be so concerned about offence but concerned about justice and what's happening to animals.

Then there was the comment about eating a sausage:

Phillip: I mean I am, I'm one of those people that you know, I'll listen to any argument but the, but the more militant you are, the more I'll back away from you.

Rochelle: Totally.

Philip: So, you know, if I, if you make me that angry, if you frighten me that much, I will eat a sausage.

All (except me): *Laughter.*

I couldn't help but wonder how Philip would react if someone said that the protesting against the killing of dogs in Asia made them want to go and eat a dog.

It's important to say, however obvious this is, that any violent threats, whether from vegans or not, are detestable and always wrong. It does, though, speak to the point I was making earlier: throughout the whole segment I was repeatedly asked how far I was willing to go and whether I agreed with meat eaters being sent death threats, accompanied by audible sighs of disgust at the threats vegans had been accused of sending, but Julie Bindel wasn't at any point asked if she condoned the threats that I, or any other vegan, have been sent.

SEEING THROUGH THE FACADE

It's important for us to recognise how much power the media and advertising have in terms of their ability to influence us as consumers, especially as they don't always promote products that are beneficial for us; after all, it wasn't that long ago that there were adverts with doctors recommending cigarettes.[19] The links between smoking and cancer had already been established, they were just not universally believed at that time and had not taken hold in a society that was reluctant to believe that smoking was dangerous, partly because it was so prevalent and normalised and partly because we had been told it was healthy. Sound familiar?

A similar thing has been documented happening with regards to climate change, with the fossil fuel lobby following in the footsteps of the tobacco industry and funding scientists and PR companies in an attempt to create doubt about the link between emissions and the climate crisis. And the same tactic of disseminating doubt is being used by the meat, dairy and egg industries as well, and to such good effect that one of Britain's best-known TV presenters actually stated live on air that he just didn't believe the information that's coming out challenging our current consumption habits. In fact, the lead researcher behind the aforementioned industry-funded study that spurred Phillip Schofield to exclaim 'bacon is back on the menu' was awarded the 2020 distinguished research award from an industry group called the American Meat Science Association (AMSA), an organisation that 'discovers, develops, and disseminates its collective meat science knowledge'.[20]

We are constantly bombarded with adverts on TV promoting happy animals and animal products. When was the last time you saw an advert promoting vegetables or fruit? When was the last time you saw an advert promoting meat, dairy or eggs? We walk into supermarkets and we see adverts with statements such as 'happy cows produce happy milk' or 'we only source meat from high welfare farms'. There is even a brand called Happy Eggs, which, when I used to eat eggs, was the one I would always buy, because I believed that the name meant that they must treat their hens with compassion. But when you consider what actually happens to egg-laying hens, it's nothing short of outrageous that a brand can call their eggs 'happy'.

Three farms (all RSPCA assured) that produce eggs for the Happy Egg Company were exposed by an investigation in early 2021, which documented dead and decomposing birds, and birds with bloody wounds and open sores.[21] In response, a spokesperson for Noble Foods, who own the Happy Egg brand, said, 'Nothing is more important to us than the safe and proper care of our hens.'[22] This is completely at odds with that fact the hens had been debeaked, had open wounds and were all going to be killed at a slaughterhouse when they were no longer profitable. In reality, an egg-laying farm is arguably the least safe place a chicken could have the misfortune of finding themselves. This sort of rhetoric from the animal-farming industries is relentless. They simultaneously complain that clearly labelled packaging for plant-based foods is misleading and then claim that animal safety is their main priority, even when there is irrefutable video evidence that this is simply not the case.

This constant repetition of statements like the one from Noble Foods plays into a concept called the illusory truth effect, which refers to the notion that when we consistently hear statements or ideas being repeated, we perceive them as being more truthful than new statements, even if they are not. Over and over we hear the same thing from these industries: farmers love their animals and always make their wellbeing a priority; we have the best standards in the world; meat, dairy and eggs are important for a balanced diet. And the list goes on. And every time we hear these statements or go into a supermarket and see a picture of a smiling farmer in a field with a statement about what a lovely life the animals are allowed to live, it becomes easier and easier for us to believe that it is true.

The advertisement of meat, eggs and dairy also directly ties into many of the ideas that were discussed in the previous chapter, as it can help perpetuate many of the prevailing attitudes that encourage us to continue consuming animal products. Presenting us with images of happy, smiling animals – such as Laughing Cow spreadable cheese – promotes the idea that they are willing participants in their exploitation and death. It immediately eases our conscience, as we presume that the product comes from a happy animal, as I did with the eggs.

In addition, some packaging depicts green pastures and farmyard buildings that evoke romanticised ideals of farming. Some brands and supermarkets have even created fake farm names, such as Tesco's 'Woodside Farms' and Lidl's 'Birchwood Farm'. By doing this, supermarkets are subtly influencing our perception of the products and creating the impression of transparency and traceability, as well as conjuring up this sentimentalised idea of farming. And yet these entirely fictitious farms actually further emphasise how untrustworthy and misleading animal product marketing really is.

However, while these are examples of disingenuous labelling and promotion, the way that companies market to children is downright immoral. There is, of course, no better example than McDonald's so-called 'Happy Meal', a product aimed at kids that uses toys and movie tie-ins to incentivise parents to buy it for their children. In reality, it's a box filled with processed cheese and processed meat (a class-one carcinogen and full of cholesterol, saturated fat and salt) that came from an animal who had their throat cut in a slaughterhouse. Yet all of this is conveniently ignored and is instead packaged in a kid-friendly way.

THE VEGAN CHICKEN KIEV

One of my favourite foods before I went vegan was a chicken kiev. When I became vegan, I had to accept that I would probably never eat one again. I thought that if there ever was a vegan chicken kiev produced, that would be a sign of how much things were changing. In fact, when I first went vegan, just the thought of being able to get vegan cheese at a regular supermarket seemed crazy. If I wanted to get vegan alternatives, I had to go to a niche organic store, which were few and far between, and even then the selection of vegan options could be lacklustre to say the least.

In the space of just a few years, everything has changed. Not only are vegan alternatives found everywhere, but their sales are increasing exponentially as well. Between 2018 and 2020, there was a 49 per cent growth in the volume of plant-based foods being consumed in the EU,[23] and in the USA sales rose by 27 per cent in 2020 alone.[24] I'm pleased to say that there are even several different brands now making vegan chicken kievs, which taste exactly the same as the ones I used to eat but without any chickens having to be killed.

However, the rise of plant-based foods hasn't been viewed positively by everyone and has led to a push back from the animal exploitation industries, which have focused on challenging the labelling of plant-based alternatives. The aforementioned bias in food marketing is even more egregious when you consider that in the EU, plant-based food companies can't legally call their plant milks 'milk', because it's deemed as being confusing and misleading to the consumer. It was even debated by the EU whether plant-based products could be called 'burgers' or 'sausages'. Thankfully, the so-called 'burger ban' wasn't passed, but it seems peculiar that a packet of 'meat-free burgers' would be seen as potentially confusing, whereas a carton of 'happy eggs' is perfectly acceptable.

Unbelievably, the 'burger ban' isn't even the most extreme example of censorship of plant-based products that the EU has attempted. Amendment 171, which the European Commission initially voted in favour of in late 2020 before it was then rejected by the European Parliament seven months later, was an attempt to go even further, making it illegal for plant-based foods to describe their products in a manner that uses familiar dairy terminology – for example, 'it's like milk', 'creamy' and 'buttery' – or even to use more directly informative descriptions, such as 'does not contain milk' and 'plant-based alternative to yoghurt', as they still contain the words 'milk' and 'yoghurt'. More concerning still, plant-based companies may have not been allowed to make comparisons between the environmental impact of their products versus dairy products, advertise their products in a way that could be interpreted as being visually similar to a dairy product – such as showing a white foam swirling into a coffee – or use typical dairy packaging, such as yoghurt pots. And the reason for all of this? Because it's confusing for consumers, who are apparently too uneducated and gullible to understand that something labelled as a 'plant-based alternative' is indeed just that. Which leads me to wonder when the EU is going to ban hot dogs for not actually containing dogs, fish fingers for not containing fingers and hamburgers for not containing ham. Which should be called pig flesh anyway.

And what about peanut butter or coconut milk? How is it that these two items have not caused the kind of consumer 'confusion' that the EU members who voted in favour of Amendment 171 claim they were trying to protect their constituents from? How many times have you bought a tin of coconut milk to then get home and be dismayed to find out that it isn't cow's milk but actually coconut milk? Never? And yet the EU wants us to believe that this is what is happening with customers when they are buying oat milk. Call me cynical, but it seems as if consumer confusion wasn't really the main motivation behind proposed legislation such as Amendment 171.

This becomes increasingly apparent when viewed alongside a study published in late 2020 that was the first of its kind to explore whether or not plant-based companies using words like 'milk' and 'meat' was actually causing confusion to consumers. The research discovered that consumers are not more likely to think that plant-based products are in fact animal products and that actually stopping plant-based companies from being able to use these words causes more confusion, as the consumers don't know what tastes the plant-based products are supposed to replicate or how they should be used.[25]

This sort of thing is not just happening in the EU. In the USA, a large number of states, including Missouri, Mississippi, Montana, South Dakota, Wyoming, Texas, Oklahoma,

Nebraska, Iowa, Colorado and Louisiana, among others, have also attempted to implement similar bans on plant-based food and cell-cultured meat labelling. Interestingly, seven of the ten biggest cattle farming states appear on that list, which is perhaps not surprising when the National Cattlemen's Beef Association's top policy priority in 2019 was addressing 'false and deceptive marketing', and they created a petition calling on the word 'meat' to be used only for animals farmed in the traditional manner.[26] This is ironic coming from an industry that uses selective breeding, artificial insemination and genetically modified crops, not to mention growth promoters, hormones and antibiotics, to maximise their profits.

It's also worth mentioning that many of these states would classify themselves as having a 'small government' approach to politics, a phrase that signifies upholding libertarian values of limited government intervention, especially in terms of public policy and private-sector regulation. Except, of course, the very opposite is true when it comes to their involvement in censoring the plant-based sector. Obviously, one of the primary reasons for this comes down to the relationship that the agricultural sector has with government and there's no better example of this than the dairy industry.

FAST FOOD AND HIT JOBS

In 1983, the US dairy industry lobbied Congress to allow them to create the National Dairy Checkoff, also known as the Dairy Promotion Program, a scheme where dairy farmers pay into a pot of money that, among other things, is then used for promotional campaigns to encourage consumers to buy more dairy products. However, while the programme is funded by dairy farmers, the federal government oversees, evaluates and approves almost every aspect of it, with United States Department of Agriculture (USDA) employees attending checkoff meetings.

The USDA is also the government organisation that writes nutritional guidelines in the USA. This is especially concerning as it means that they are not only responsible for the creation of adverts promoting dairy consumption but they also advise people on how much dairy to consume in the first place. Which could possibly explain why the USDA still recommends adults consume three servings of dairy a day, while the Canadian ideal food plate has removed dairy as a food group altogether, and even though it is still listed as a protein source, there are no recommendations for how much to consume or that you even need to consume it at all.

To make matters worse, Dairy Management Inc. (DMI), which is funded by the USDA-managed dairy checkoff programme, works with schools and fast-food chains to increase overall dairy consumption. For example, DMI has worked with McDonald's to increase the size of cheddar cheese slices by more than 30 per cent in some of their items and with Pizza Hut to add 25 per cent more cheese to their pan pizza. They also created a pizza with Domino's that contained as much as two thirds of a day's maximum recommended amount of saturated fat.[27] So the government department that creates the nutritional guidelines and advises people how to eat healthily also works with the farming industries to promote their products and get more of them sold in fast-food chains and restaurants.

It's not just the USDA's involvement in the dairy checkoff programme that is alarming. In 2014, US company Hampton Creek, now called Just, was generating a significant amount of interest in their plant-based egg and mayonnaise substitutes. This concerned the American Egg Board (AEB), a US government appointed agricultural body that, as shown in emails acquired through a freedom of information request, viewed Hampton Creek as being a 'major threat'.[28] Consequently, they launched a concerted effort to attack the company, including trying to get the supermarket chain Whole Foods to stop selling their products and advising Unilever (who produce Hellmann's mayonnaise) on how to build a lawsuit against Hampton Creek for false advertising.

One of the heads of the USDA also joined the attack on Hampton Creek and suggested that the AEB should contact the government Food and Drug Administration (FDA) to see if they could help with their concerns. And if that wasn't shady enough, the freedom of information obtained emails revealing that the head of the AEB was involved in a conversation where an executive vice president of an AEB member organisation said in reference to Hampton Creek CEO Josh Tetrick, 'Can we pool our money and put a hit on him?'[29] There was even an email from the executive vice president of the AEB offering 'to contact some of my old buddies in Brooklyn to pay Mr Tetrick a visit'.[30]

These disturbing emails and the potential that the AEB had used funds illegally in their anti-Hampton Creek campaign were placed under investigation. However, it was led by the USDA, the same government department that had appointed the members of the AEB and that was itself implicated by the allegations. Perhaps unsurprisingly, then, they found no criminal wrongdoing and decided that the emails were sent in jest.[31] I wonder if the USDA would have felt the same if the tables had been turned and Hampton Creek executives had been sending emails about paying for hits on members of USDA-appointed agency employees?

Meat industry lobbying further contributes to the problem of government and industry collusion, with ten of the biggest meat companies in the USA spending $26 million in the past 20 years alone on political campaigns and over $100 million on lobbying in general. When the amount spent on lobbying is viewed as a percentage of the company's overall revenue, Tyson has spent double what oil company Exxon has spent on political campaigns. They were also revealed to be funding organisations that actively work to minimise the connection between animal farming and climate change.[32]

This industry and government collaboration isn't a uniquely American situation, though. In the UK, during the Covid-19 pandemic, the Department for the Environment, Food and Rural Affairs (DEFRA) spent half a million pounds of taxpayers' money on a promotional campaign for the dairy industry.[33] This at a time when charities were struggling to provide food to the most vulnerable people and the NHS was overwhelmed. DEFRA spent more than double what the Agriculture and Horticulture Development Board (AHDB) spent on their campaign, even though one of the primary functions of the AHDB is to fund promotional campaigns on behalf of the farmers who pay the levy. Imagine the uproar if the UK government funded advertising campaigns for plant-based products and tried to get people to drink oat milk.

The AHDB also co-developed the UK's national dietary guidelines alongside Public Health England.[34] Why is a lobby group that is funded by farmers and exists to best serve their interests also a co-developer of our nutritional guidelines? The AHDB are also a 'sustaining member' (meaning they donate regularly) of the British Nutrition Association, who are another organisation involved in the creation of government dietary guidelines.[35]

Back in 2019, Michael Gove, who was at that time the minister in charge of DEFRA, also said at the National Farmers' Union conference that 'dairy farmers deserve protection from activists who would undermine their work'[36] and that he was an 'enthusiastic supporter' of the FebruDairy campaign, the one founded by the person who liked a tweet about shooting vegans. Imagine what the reaction would be if the head of DEFRA stated that they were an enthusiastic supporter of Veganuary. But why do dairy farmers deserve public support but oat farmers who produce oat milk don't?

SOY BOYS AND FRAGILE MASCULINITY

Of course, media and advertising campaigns aren't just about promoting the consumption of animal products but are also significant factors in shaping our perception of meat-eating. For example, there is a very prevalent idea that to be a real man you have to eat animal flesh and that by going vegan you are somehow emasculating yourself. This is something that I have encountered first-hand, with people calling me a 'soy boy' for being vegan. So where does this idea come from?

In some ways, it can be traced back to our nomadic roots, when it is generally thought that the men hunted and the women gathered. However, there is evidence of those roles in fact being less gender divided within some hunter-gatherer communities. That said, if we try to excuse men eating meat by saying it's because they used to be hunters, we're misunderstanding our ancestors, as for them the act of killing an animal wasn't the point – it was an act of provision. The fact that men hunted was secondary to the fact that hunting ensured communities could survive. If the idea is that eating meat is manly because men used to be hunters, then really the conclusion should be that providing for your community and looking after those around you is what makes you a man. In those terms, the idea that meat-eating is masculine is farcical, as the modern-day consumption of meat negatively impacts those around us, whether by increasing the risk of pandemics or being a significant contributor to the climate crisis.

Plus, it's much too simplistic to point to our nomadic days to justify our behaviour thousands of years later. The truth is that this attitude about masculinity and meat-eating is more closely linked to how animal products are marketed and advertised. For instance, companies will often heavily sexualise the marketing of meat products, with campaigns from companies such as Carl's Jr, Burger King, Subway and many more using imagery of women to sell their products to a male audience. Alternatively, meat companies will depict animal products as being eaten by men, with taglines such as 'Feed the Man' being used to promote Ginsters products[37] or 'Man Up' in an advert promoting a new Carl's Jr burger.[38] There was also Burger King's 'Eat Like a Man' commercial,[39] in which a guy sang about not wanting to eat 'chick food', and the 'Guys Love Bacon' campaign from Taco Bell.[40] These companies have for decades reinforced the message that red meat in particular is what men eat, so it's no wonder that this idea has become so prevalent throughout society.

All of this advertising has led to some interesting social science, though. For example, a study from the University of Hawaii found that men routinely incorporate more red meat into their diet to reassure themselves when they feel their masculinity is under threat.[41] And there can be no better demonstration of this than when Fox News host Jesse Watters ate a steak live on television in front of a social psychologist who had come on to discuss the perceived link between eating meat and masculinity.[42] In what can only be described as an astounding display of irony, Watters genuinely thought that he was hilariously dismissing her work while actually validating the very point she was making: some men who feel the need to assert their masculinity, or who feel their masculinity is being threatened, will use red meat as a means to make themselves feel more manly.

Another reason for this perceived relationship between meat and masculinity is the fact that meat is seen as a power symbol and a sign of prosperity and wealth. Our level of meat consumption in the West has only been this high for a very short period of time, coinciding with a significant period of societal progression and advancement. Consequently, we perceive unrestrained meat consumption as being a product of social modernity and symbolising the end of food scarcity and rationing, which was the paradigm in the early twentieth century before the rise of industrial agriculture and intensive animal farming.

This idea of meat being viewed as a power symbol was shown in a paper published in the journal *Appetite*.[43] The researchers collected a group of participants from a range of backgrounds and found that those who were lower on the economic scale had a greater preference for meat than those higher up it. The researchers concluded that this was 'likely because people see meat as substitutable for status', so wanting to eat meat was a reflection of how the participants felt about their own circumstances in life. Studies such as this one also provide interesting explanations as to why fast-food chains, which have been shown to be five times more prevalent in lower-income areas of many cities in the UK,[44] are often the same companies that most heavily perpetuate the idea of meat being a male status symbol.

A huge issue with this mindset is that it can dissuade men who want to stop eating meat from doing so. A piece of research presented at the Royal Geographical Society showed that men find it difficult to choose the vegan option when in public with other men and that those who reduced their intake of animal protein even reported experiencing social isolation among their male friends.[45] The researchers stated that the men perceived the need for social permission to choose a meat-free option. There is, however, an obvious irony in the fact that meat is supposedly seen as a sign of strength and status but is being eaten because some men are too afraid to make a change in front of other men.

This point highlights the wider fallacy of the perceived link between meat and masculinity. Those who say they eat meat because it makes them manly are the ones who are most conscious about their masculinity in the first place. If men were truly comfortable with their masculinity, they wouldn't feel the need to prove anything to anyone. In the same way that meat was used as a substitute for a perceived lack of status, the same must also be true for masculinity.

We've talked about how social pressure heavily influences our decision making. So combining social pressure with a man's fear of his masculinity being questioned creates an incredibly challenging prospect for men who might want to become vegan. The idea that men in these situations are so susceptible to social conformity or pressure might seem hyperbolic; however, the famous Milgram experiment further emphasises just how challenging the act of going against what you are being told by those around you can be.

In 1963, Stanley Milgram carried out a study to explore the relationship between obedience to authority and personal conscience. He demonstrated that the participants in the experiment were willing to administer increasingly strong 'electric shocks' to a knowing participant in the study (the shocks were in fact fake). Milgram explained this behaviour by concluding that in certain situations people can sometimes enter what is known as the agent state, where they allow other people to direct their actions and try to pass off any responsibility for these actions by blaming the person whom they are obeying.

Although Milgram's experiment was more specifically about the effect of authority figures, in an attempt to explain how people who worked in concentration camps were able to carry out their orders, a related dynamic can play out in social situations. Men encounter increasing pressure from their peers if they seem to want to choose a plant-based option, to the point where it becomes easier for the person to choose the meat option but psychologically distance themselves from the responsibility of the action by blaming it on the person who is making them obedient.

This phenomenon is something that meat, dairy and egg advertisers are very much aware of and use in their campaigns, with adverts such as the aforementioned Burger King's 'Eat Like a Man' advert featuring hundreds of men singing 'I am man' as they talk about eating a beef burger, which not only creates a fabricated sense of peer pressure from hundreds of fictional male characters but creates a false idea of gendered foods through the use of imperative and authoritative language: 'Wave tofu bye bye. Now it's the Whopper beef I reach. I will eat this meat.'

Often without us realising, our preconceptions about different foods and what they symbolise are dictated by a variety of external factors. In the case of men, the narrative around red meat and masculinity has been moulded through decades of advertising that attempts to reinforce this idea, although in reality it's not substantiated by anything meaningful or relevant.

A VERY INCONVENIENT TRUTH

It is incredibly frustrating how underreported the impact of animal agriculture is, and it's certainly not down to a lack of studies to report on. It can feel like an uphill battle trying to raise awareness about these issues when they are so often ignored by the media, or when the media instead pushes sensationalist stories, such as the vegan dying while climbing Everest. I find myself having to regularly deal with arguments that people have read online and haven't properly researched themselves, whether it's that tofu is destroying the Amazon and is filled with oestrogen or that vegans are actually responsible for killing more animals. And did I mention that a vegan died climbing Everest?

Perhaps even more frustrating is how readily information about the impact of animal farming is disregarded by people as being propaganda (probably because they don't see it being discussed enough in the media). But this is nothing new. Broader coverage of the consequences of animal farming has historically been very infrequent, with one study that looked at 16 leading US newspapers from 2005 to 2008 identifying 4,500 articles about climate change but only 2.4 per cent of those mentioning the contribution of animal agriculture to the crisis.[46] Another study that looked at coverage from 2006 to 2018 in four major media organisations, two in the UK and two in the USA, discovered that only 4 per cent of the 114,000 articles that mentioned climate change also mentioned animal agriculture.[47]

This lack of coverage was in spite of the fact that the UN's landmark report on animal farming and the environment, called 'Livestock's Long Shadow', was released in 2006.[48] The report outlined the need to acknowledge animal farming as a major contributor to the climate crisis but, as these studies show, that didn't happen. This in turn had an impact on public opinion, with a 2020 government survey on members of the UK public showing that only 22 per cent of people perceived agriculture as contributing a 'great deal' to the climate crisis.[49]

A huge part of the problem is that the animal agriculture industries perpetuate misinformation and create confusion in the eyes of the consumer. A 2021 investigation into ten of the biggest meat industry organisations in the world, which analysed hundreds of documents and statements by the companies, revealed that the meat industry is copying what the tobacco industry used to do and the fossil fuel industry continues to do – create confusion and doubt. They were shown to be attempting to downplay the impact that animal products have on the environment or questioning the efficacy of plant-based diets, often by funding their own studies that they then give to the press via their PR teams. They were also shown to be creating their own sustainability labels and guidelines to greenwash their products.

The report also criticised the media's role in presenting many of the meat industry's fallacies without scrutinising them, stating that journalists were 'struggling' to mediate the discussion between the meat industry PR and the scientific literature on the impact of animal farming. A Harvard Law School policy fellow stated, 'If you have virtual consensus on one side and a few people over here, many of whom received funding from the meat industry, that should be reported. It shouldn't be seen as two equal interlocutors presenting equally valid opposing opinions.'[50]

That being said, in the past several years it seems as if things have been slowly changing, especially in the advertising space, where there have been an increasing number of adverts promoting plant-based alternatives – although these adverts normally provoke a very abrupt reaction from the animal-farming industries. Case in point: an advert from Tesco promoting meatless sausages caused an uproar from the farming community. It featured a young girl coming home from school and telling her father, 'Daddy, I don't want to eat animals any more,' to which the father tells the viewers, 'I bloomin' love my meat. But not as much as I love my little girl.' The National Farmers' Union responded by attacking the advert for 'demonising meat as a food group' and said that it had 'caused significant distress for British farmers'.[51]

Rather farcically, the NFU even criticised the BBC for a promotional Christmas advert, where in one scene an animated cartoon turkey is depicted wearing a knitted jumper that says 'I love vegans' on it. The vice president of the union said it showed an 'agenda against livestock farming'.[52]

Although responses such as these might seem ludicrous, the animal farming community is actually being deadly serious. For years, meat, dairy and egg companies have monopolised the advertising space, creating narratives and ideas about animal consumption and perpetuating preconceptions in order to continue selling their products. This is ultimately why they react with such hostility to plant-based advertising and anything that contradicts the narrative they have dominated for decades. After all, they know how powerful advertising can be, and for the first time they are beginning to see it being used to disrupt their industries.

BELIEVING THE FACTS

Ultimately, the changing landscape of the advertising world and of consumer attitudes shows that while there has been historical media and institutional bias in protecting the interests of animal agriculture, that bias hasn't been able to stop the gradual shifts that are occurring. Previous generations didn't have access to the information that is available to us today – we are now able to look at both sides of the debate and apply some important scrutiny to the information that we had little choice but to take at face value in the past.

For too long, meat industry boards, lobby groups and industry-funded PR campaigns have dominated the narrative but the facade of animal farming is slowly beginning to crumble. The world's most-renowned and highly regarded scientific organisations and institutions are repeatedly warning us about the dangers, both global and individual, of animal farming, and the reality of what animals are forced to endure is becoming not only better understood but increasingly harder to ignore.

Importantly, issues that were once rarely if ever discussed are becoming a more familiar part of the conversation. As consumers, we are now able to see how biases are being perpetuated and how they are meant to drive our behaviours and attitudes. Because of this, we can empower ourselves, and indeed each other, to instead make informed decisions with a broader understanding of what the reality of animal farming and the damage it causes actually is.

The American author Seth Godin once said, 'Facts are irrelevant. What matters is what the consumer believes.' This is the philosophy the animal agriculture industries have relied on for decades, tricking consumers into believing things that are simply not true. However, consumers are now beginning to believe the facts, and for animal agriculture, nothing could be worse.

9.

TALKING ABOUT VEGANISM

Before going vegan, I had a variety of worries: where would I get my protein? Was it possible to live without cheese? What if I never learned to like tofu? But none of these concerns turned out to be the most challenging part of choosing veganism – after all, protein is easy to obtain on a plant-based diet, and I soon found out that there actually are good vegan cheeses out there.

What I, and most vegans I have spoken to, have found to be the most difficult aspect of rejecting animal products is the strain it puts on your relationships with other people, especially family. The food side of things is easy – in fact, I enjoy a wider variety of foods and flavours now than I ever did before I was vegan. And the nutrients aspect is not a problem because, as I've shown, all it takes is a little research and you can easily obtain everything you need to not only be healthy but to thrive. The cravings go as well: the cheese I once thought was irresistible I now see as nothing more than a product of exploitation and suffering.

But I often say that I would rather have a conversation with a dairy farmer than a member of my own family about veganism. Since going vegan, I have been to more livestock auctions than I have family get-togethers, more slaughterhouses than I have birthdays and meals. I have spent more time on farms than at my family's houses. The prospect of being stopped by a farmer is apparently less daunting than my mum sitting down and saying, 'Well, Edward, the thing about veganism is . . .'

I don't say this as an indictment of my own family – far from it. It's a product of my fear of confrontation with those I love. Entering into a conversation with a family member about veganism could lead to an argument or a sense of disappointment that those who I most desperately want to be vegan will defend meat-eating so ardently to my face. To think of animals being abused and killed while listening to my own family defend why they eat meat is something that fills me with great sorrow.

LIFE LESSONS FROM AN OSPREY

One of the reasons I find it so difficult to talk to my loved ones about veganism is that my family were actually a great influence on me becoming vegan in the first place. As I've said, we would go on regular walks and trips out to the countryside when I was younger, and we went on an almost annual trip to Scotland, the purpose of which was to go on lots of hikes. During our trips, we would always stay in a cabin, nestled in a forested area, secluded and away from any main roads. There, seeing deer and other majestic wild animals was an everyday occurrence.

In one of my clearest and perhaps fondest memories of one these holidays in Scotland, I remember standing with my family at dusk watching as a cow gave birth to a calf in a field. As we looked on, we remarked how beautiful new life and birth was and how lucky we were to have witnessed such a thing. Yet no doubt during that same day we would have consumed cow's milk, cheese and cow-flesh products – an almost excoriating irony considering the very species of animal we were proclaiming admiration and affection for was also likely being digested in our stomachs at that very same time.

On another day, my mum and I went out for a stroll together through the woodlands around the property. As we were walking, a deer suddenly ran out in front of us. We were both in awe of the animal and struck by the way they moved with such grace and majesty. I think of this moment now and juxtapose it with eating venison and my family making the joke, 'Why don't we eat venison more? It's a little bit deer.'

These two moments summarise so much about the hypocrisy of how we live – the fact that many of us are in awe of animals and wouldn't want to kill them ourselves but are instead happy to pay for someone else to do the killing for us, as that way we can pretend we are less accountable for the act of taking life.

This hypocrisy was also revealed by the fishing experiences I had as a child. We would go to a lake where fish were bred specifically to be caught by anglers. Every time we were there, we would always catch and release, even though we could club the fish to death if we wanted to. I very vividly remember watching as another fisherman held a fish down on a wooden block and proceeded to club them to death, repeatedly hitting them, the fish desperately flapping as they were both suffocating and being bludgeoned at the same time. The violence of that moment really struck me. Even though I was fishing too and had no right to judge, it was an act of barbarism that I simply couldn't understand. What disturbed me even more about this situation was that it wasn't an exercise in survival – it was a leisurely day out. This person was clubbing the fish to death because it was enjoyable for him, a recreational activity.

On reflection, what is even more bewildering about those experiences of fishing is that although my family would never kill the fish, we would go to the shop at the lake afterwards and buy rainbow trout that had already been killed but had not yet been gutted or butchered. We would then take them home and gut and butcher them ourselves. We would catch and release these animals and then buy them whole in the shop to cook and eat, but we wouldn't do the actual killing. It was never our hands that held the terrified fish down, nor was it our clubs that were brought down onto their heads. Is it not strange that if a child threw a rock at a cat, society would view that child as antisocial or exhibiting violent tendencies, but encouraging a child to go out on a family fishing trip, or to go out hunting to shoot a deer, is a wholesome family bonding activity? The violence is still violence; the end result is still causing suffering to an animal and taking their life.

In Scotland, one of the activities we engaged in most often was watching ospreys at Loch Garten nature reserve; in fact, we were earnest members of the Royal Society for the Protection of Birds (RSPB). At the nature reserve, you could watch a webcam showing what the ospreys were up to and learn about them as individuals, as the centre had given each osprey a name and provided information about their specific personality traits. We would see the ospreys go about their normal activities, enthralled as we witnessed events such as a new male osprey invading the nest and kicking out Odin (one of the male ospreys) and his mate EJ's eggs. It was like a version of *The Truman Show* but specifically for ospreys.

I now have a huge amount of admiration for the fact my mum and stepdad became so emotionally invested in the lives of these ospreys, and even though I wasn't as interested as they were when I was younger, I think these experiences had a larger impact on me than perhaps I initially realised. The fact that I was taught from a young age to acknowledge the behavioural variation of non-human animals, as well as understanding them to be complex individuals with rich personalities, no doubt helped lay the foundations for me to acknowledge, as I do now, the irrational and inconsistent mentality we have towards different species of animals. Furthermore, from those experiences of being a passive voyeur, I recognised that to gain my respect and admiration non-human animals need to offer me nothing in return. Yet, for many of us living in urban environments, the only animals we outwardly care about are the animals who have enriched our lives, such as the dogs we have in our homes, an almost tacit belief that they are worthy of moral consideration because they have formed a mutual relationship with us.

Perhaps this is why I find my family's somewhat disinterested attitude to veganism even more upsetting than I would anyone else's. I have a memory from when I was a child of my stepdad staring despondently out of the window because a dog that belonged to one of his relatives, and who he cared about deeply, had just died. He always had a very strong connection with the dog, and to him it was like losing a family member. The way that we react and mourn when pets die speaks volumes about how we perceive our relationship with other animals, as well as our ability to empathise with them. If only we showed a fraction of that same empathy to all the other animals we so flippantly disregard.

Unfortunately, I also have experience from the more upsetting end of the spectrum of how loved ones can react around vegans. One time, upon hearing that my mum was coming to visit me for the day, a family member told her to eat a ham sandwich in front of me to taunt me, something that even now, several years later, still upsets me.

Thankfully, my mum didn't do that and we instead had an entirely vegan lunch at a restaurant nearby. The thing is, that family member is a compassionate and kind person, and

I am very fond of them. But there is something about being around vegans that can make people act very differently to how they normally would. I have spoken to countless vegans who have cried as they recounted stories of their family members secretly putting meat in their food, mocking them or shouting at them. Family members doing the kinds of things you would expect a school bully to do, except they're this person's parent or sibling. And all because they don't want to eat products that come from animal exploitation. I have so much sympathy for young vegans who are not vocal activists but instead just people who have made the decision that they want to reduce as much as possible the suffering they cause to animals. For that to create a hostile or tumultuous relationship with their parents, such that it brings that person to tears when they describe it, is unconscionable to me. However, it is clear that many vegans feel a great sense of fear about being rejected by their family members or causing rifts in their relationships.

WALKING THE TIGHTROPE

I do, however, understand why parents might not always take to their child becoming vegan with the kind of eagerness that the child hopes or expects. One of the roles of a parent is to raise their children with values and morals – to make them a good person. So, from the perspective of a parent, when their child says to them that they are becoming vegan because it's not morally justifiable to exploit animals, it could be seen as the child implying that they have been raised badly. Of course, that's not what's intended, but, subconsciously, the parent could feel like they are being personally criticised by their child's decision. It is understandable, therefore, why a parent might be defensive or even angry at their child living in a way that they perceive as being an implicit criticism of their parenting and lifestyle. I think it requires a great deal of humility for a parent to then take an active interest in their child's veganism and engage in a positive manner, and even more so if they then adopt a vegan lifestyle themselves.

The issue of disconnection from one's parents is, however, merely one example that illustrates a wider scope of problems related to social disconnection when one becomes vegan. You see good people around you engaging in acts that perpetuate huge amounts of suffering and violence. Witnessing those you care about causing suffering to others can be extremely challenging. Pop culture and the media so often reinforce the idea that good and evil are clear cut, that an individual's character is not as complex as it is in reality. But, in many ways, going vegan reinforces the moral complexity of real life, as most people engaging with these industries are not bad people. In fact, many are among some of the nicest, most compassionate and caring people you are likely to meet. Yet despite their kindness, every time they buy animal products, they are paying for someone else to inflict pain and suffering on other sentient beings – things they would never want to do themselves, precisely because they are compassionate and caring people.

A few years ago, my grandparents celebrated their 60th wedding anniversary, and they arranged a huge family get-together to celebrate the occasion. The only problem was that the meal consisted mainly of animal products. I couldn't face the prospect of sitting around several dozen people eating the remains of animals who had died so that we could celebrate the coming together of our family and the 60-year union of my grandparents. It didn't seem right that a day of celebration should be marred by the suffering of others.

Our most joyous days of celebration and ritual are often marked by the mass death of others. We celebrate Christmas and Thanksgiving by confining tens of millions of turkeys in windowless barns, where many of them die of organ failure, the ones who survive then being taken to slaughterhouses. We celebrate Easter by killing newborn lambs so we can eat their legs and have a wonderful day of celebration, talking about how the remains of a baby animal are so tender and juicy.

We do the same for sporting events as well, with the Super Bowl in the USA being celebrated with the consumption of 1.35 billion chicken wings during the course of the weekend, which means that around 700 million chickens are killed just for a sporting event,[1] with a staggering 99.9 per cent of them being raised on a factory farm,[2] suffering immensely before being forced into crates and taken to slaughterhouses. It is estimated that this number of wings is enough to circle the Earth three times.[3] But most of the people who are consuming these wings are not bad people and would be horrified at the prospect of having to take an active part in this process.

When it came to the anniversary party, I thought about my grandparents – the most gentle, kind and loving people – celebrating such a wonderful event by eating the remains of animals who had lived lives of abject suffering. To me, that juxtaposition of celebration, union and love with misery, torture and death was one that I couldn't rationalise. I decided, therefore, that I didn't want to sit and eat with my family during the anniversary celebration and that I would instead join them afterwards. I know this might seem extreme, but if I had been invited to an event and saw the menu included a starter of Labrador tartar, followed by grilled cat with a gravy made from the fat of a whale and a cheesecake made with gelatine from the boiled skin, tendons and bones of a husky for dessert, wouldn't the normal reaction be to voice some sort of objection?

I realise that in not joining my family for the meal I was further contributing to my own familial disconnection. However, the thought of my implicit condoning of animal exploitation by normalising the act through my participation at the event was something that I could not accept from a moral perspective. This is the balancing act that vegans face: we either voice our objection and get labelled as extremist, militant, awkward or abnormal, or we stay silent and smile through the image of a cow having their throat cut that passes through our minds as we watch our loved ones bite into beef burgers. We either feel like we are betraying our morals out of fear of causing upset or find ourselves being labelled as preachy, forceful vegan extremists.

RATIONALISING THE REACTIONS OF OTHERS

The problem, however, goes further than this. Many vegans who attempt to keep it to themselves still end up on the receiving end of the ire of someone within their social circle. Even when I have gone to events or parties with the intention of not having any discussion about my lifestyle, someone who knows me will either bring up my veganism or I'll be offered something to eat that I have to politely decline, which will then create the kind of conversation that I was trying to avoid.

On one occasion, I was having a good time and minding my own business at a party when someone I had never met before found out I was a vegan and took it upon themselves to tell me repeatedly that lions eat other animals, each time becoming more impatient and incredulous. I sat there sipping on my drink, explaining that we shouldn't base our morality on the actions of wild animals while trying to work out if I had stayed long enough to be able to leave without seeming rude.

To further reiterate the significance of food and personal connections, a recent poll from the UK showed that around half of Brits are now worried about catering to everyone's dietary needs when they are hosting a barbecue.[4] This might seem a bit inconsequential, but it speaks volumes about the importance of food when it comes to socialising. In fact, food is an integral part of the relationships we have with others, and when someone goes vegan and no longer wants to eat at the same restaurant they have always celebrated their wedding anniversary at, or doesn't want to eat at the same place they always do with their friends, or doesn't want to eat the food their friends have bought for a barbecue, the dynamics of our most important relationships are altered in ways that haven't been mutually agreed. We find so much comfort and reassurance in these small things. They create unity and foster connections, so even though the moral importance of going vegan far outweighs these social stresses, they shouldn't be denied or their significance diminished or ignored.

These social strains can lead to people being mocked from within their friendship circles or by their families, because on a subconscious level there can often exist some level of resentment or fear of a lack of control. People often want to re-establish a sense of being in the right or to persuade the person to no longer be vegan, in an attempt to return everything to how it used to be. It's not that these actions come from a bad place necessarily; it's more a result of insecurity and fear that their relationships are now going to be different, that aspects of their lives that they used to enjoy so much are not going to be the same or even that the vegans in their lives might encourage them to start to question their own actions.

THE MEAT PARADOX

It is of course true that flesh-eating still enjoys a dominant status but veganism is an increasing threat to the normalisation of the industrialised killing and consumption of other species. Even so, the levels of animosity directed at vegans can be startling. In fact, research has shown that only drug addicts face the same degree of stigma as vegans, with male vegans who have gone vegan for ethical reasons being viewed the most negatively.[5] This seems strange considering almost everyone is against animal cruelty; it doesn't therefore make sense that one of the most reviled groups of people in society is the one that is actively trying to reduce the amount of cruelty caused to animals.

Social psychologist Dr Hank Rothgerber believes that a lot of the animosity towards vegans comes from the fact that 'we live in an era today, at least in the Western world, where there's more and more evidence, more and more arguments, and more and more books about how eating meat is bad . . . So what I'm looking at is, how do people rationalise that, and still feel like they're a good person?'[6]

One of the most common things that people say to vegans online is that they are about to go and eat a steak, or a piece of bacon, or even that they are currently eating an animal product as they are typing. What is most baffling about this behaviour is how much power people assign to these sorts of comments, as if they truly believe that telling a vegan about someone consuming an animal product will upset them more than anything else. But we all live in a non-vegan world, so vegans are surrounded by these products and people consuming them all the time. Part of the problem seems to be that eating animal products is so normalised that people don't view it as an ideology or as a belief system – or even as an active choice that they make. Psychologist Dr Melanie Joy coined the term 'carnism' to describe the prevailing ideology of animal-product consumption, which she defines as being an invisible belief system that is supported by a variety of defence mechanisms and mostly unchallenged assumptions. One of these defence systems is something that is often referred to as the 'meat paradox',[7] meaning the juxtaposition of one's values with one's actions when it comes to animals – although this should really be called the 'animal product paradox', as of course the same ethical problems and subsequent psychological defence mechanisms are still prevalent when it comes to dairy and egg consumption as well.

A fascinating example of this idea is that farmers love their animals and want only the best for them, while still profiting from sending them to a slaughterhouse to be killed. It is undeniably a contradiction to claim to love someone who you intend to kill for money. However, this is one of the most ardent beliefs among those who eat animals: that the animals they eat are treated with love and compassion, and that they even have their lives taken needlessly and against their will in a 'kind' way.

Denying the intelligence and consciousness of the animals that we deem to be 'food' is one of the other interesting aspects of the meat paradox. In 2010, a study was conducted with college students in which they were randomly given either beef jerky or cashews to eat.[8] They were then asked to judge the intellectual and cognitive capabilities of certain animals and their moral importance. The results found that those who had been given the beef jerky deemed cows to have a lower intellectual ability and a diminished mental capacity to experience things such as suffering and pain, and they expressed less moral concern for animals when compared to those who had eaten the cashews.

When it comes to the meat paradox, our brains are constantly working to rationalise our behaviours, even to the point that our subconscious view of animals fluctuates based on whether or not we have just eaten animal products. This is why trying to communicate with people about veganism while they are eating or shortly after they have finished is probably one of the least effective times to do so, and why, if you are not vegan, you feel most defensive around the times that you are eating. This is not, of course, surprising. We have hardwired ourselves to deal with the feelings of discomfort that arise when our morality is questioned – there are many examples of this beyond veganism too.

The beef jerky study suggests a potential reason why people might make the point of eating animals in front of vegans, or telling them they are going to eat animal products as a result of being around them – they subconsciously connect the concept of eating animal products with a reduction in their feelings of guilt. So, if a vegan has caused them to feel guilty or uncomfortable, making a reference to eating an animal product is a psychological defence to try to diminish those feelings.

This helps to explain why being around a vegan can bring out such abrupt and often uncharacteristic responses. It also provides a possible explanation for why my family member told my mum to eat the ham sandwich in front of me. Being confronted with veganism reaffirms that what, or who, we eat is an active choice, and suddenly the consumption of meat comes with the label of being an 'animal eater' as opposed to just being 'normal'. Consequently, vegans make the status quo feel that bit more uncomfortable, eroding the sense of safety provided by the bandwagon effect. The comedian David Mitchell summarised this when he said, 'The thing that's annoying about there suddenly being a lot of them [vegans] is the nagging suspicion that they might be right. When there were hardly any vegans, I hardly ever had to think about that.'[9]

This form of rationalisation makes it much easier for us to understand the often confusing reaction of our parents or others around us when we go vegan. So, when it comes to the issue of social disconnection and veganism, it is in reality a double-edged sword: vegans fear losing their connections with friends and family while, at the same time, those within a vegan's social circles feel as if their relationship is being changed against their will and their belief systems are being called into question by virtue of engaging with a vegan.

It is no wonder, then, that there can be so much tension and even conflict in the interpersonal relationships of vegans and non-vegans. It is easy for us to take situations and reactions at face value but, as with most things, what's really going on beneath the surface can be a lot more complicated than meets the eye.

A deeper understanding of what drives human behaviour is liberating as a vegan, as it can ensure that we don't see the actions of those we love as evidence that they are bad people. Whether we consciously think about it or not, our actions are driven by a multitude of factors. That can mean that a meat eater's opinion of veganism is not necessarily their true view of what it means to be vegan but instead a reflection of the complicated psychological processes that they are undergoing to rationalise an action that, for the majority of us, goes against some of our most intrinsic values.

THE FEAR OF DISCONNECTION

In the end, I know that I shouldn't avoid discussions about veganism with my family for ever, but finding a way to navigate the at times exceedingly complex psychological and emotional mechanisms that cause these disconnections is daunting. It is obvious that the reason family and friends are the hardest to be around is because we care so deeply about these people, and the fear of causing a rift or creating a barrier can at times have the opposite effect and lead to an even bigger rift or barrier forming. We allow the fear of change or disconnection to make us act in an uncharacteristic way, whether that's taunting a vegan relative with a piece of meat or calling our non-vegan friend an animal abuser.

Ultimately, we need to create healthy dialogue and discussion and recognise that the reason our relationships with those close to us can become strained is because they are of the most importance to us. I often wonder whether it was right of me to not eat with my family during my grandparents' 60th wedding anniversary. Perhaps in the pursuit of upholding my own principles I inadvertently perpetuated the self-righteous reputation that vegans are often viewed as having. Or maybe my attempt to take a principled stand encouraged some members of my family to reflect on their own values, revealing to them, even subconsciously, their own cognitive dissonance. Either way, whether it was the right thing to do or not, one thing for sure is that it further highlighted the complexity and challenges that veganism can place on our most important relationships.

I wonder, though, if I sat down with my family and heard my mum say, 'Well, Edward, the thing about veganism is . . .' would it be as daunting as I initially feared? One day I'll have to drum up the courage to find out.

CREATING MORE EFFECTIVE CONVERSATIONS ABOUT VEGANISM

While I have often shied away from having conversations with my family about veganism, I have spent the past six years having many conversations about veganism with almost anyone else that I could. I've spoken with many farmers from different industries and different countries, cowboys in Texas, hunters, slaughterhouse workers, journalists, TV presenters, academics and everyday meat-eaters. I've spoken with people sympathetic towards veganism and people who are less so. Through these conversations, I've found certain things that can really help to create constructive and healthy dialogue – not just with people we have never met before, but also with those who are the most important in our lives as well.

1. Be well educated and prepared

Before engaging in a discussion about veganism, it is important take some time to try to learn some of the basics – as you have just done by reading this book. Most people use the same arguments when talking about veganism, so take some time to learn how to respond to some of the main points covered in this book as well as any others you've come across before.

With loved ones, the conversation can often become about where to get nutrients from or how the cooking is going to change, so pre-emptively research and find out where vegans can get protein, iron, calcium and omega-3 – the main nutrients that we think we need from animal products. Also, look up vegan recipes online, as there are vegan versions of almost every meal you can think of. It can be a good idea to offer to cook some meals for your family and, if you are not usually the person who does the food shopping, to buy in some of the vegan substitutes yourself so that your loved ones can try them without feeling like they have to spend money on something they don't want or might not like.

2. Ask questions

One of the most valuable techniques for creating effective conversations is to ask questions. The point is not to force one's own beliefs on the other participants in the conversation; instead, it is a means by which all participants can work cooperatively to better understand each other's views and values. Through asking questions we can encourage people to understand their position better through prompting introspection. It also ensures that those with whom you are speaking are not passive listeners but instead are active agents in the conversation and feel like they are not having points of view imposed on them.

One of the best things about asking questions is that it can stop someone from feeling like they are being judged while also making sure that the conversation addresses the importance of veganism.

3. Listen

Conversations can often become frustratingly heated when it feels like the other person isn't listening or is simply talking past us, so make sure to take the time to listen to what the other person is saying. A great way of showing that you are listening is to repeat things the person you are speaking to has said. You can do this by clarifying their position back to them. For example, 'I can completely understand where you're coming from. I used to eat meat because it tastes nice as well. But do you think that taste has higher value than life?'

Alternatively, you can validate what someone says before then asking a question or showing them why what they have said is wrong. For example, 'It's completely understandable that you would think that we need to eat meat for protein; after all, we've been told this our whole lives. But do you think it's possible to get protein from plant foods?'

4. Watch body language

In many ways, our body language and the way we say something is just as important as what we actually say. Lots of us have little idiosyncratic behaviours we adopt without realising – for example, when I get in a confrontation with someone, I have a habit of pointing with my right index finger, so if I feel myself getting irritated, I have to be conscious of how my body language is changing as a result. Make sure to seem open and relaxed and try not to point or clench. A great way of doing this is to keep your palms open and your arms to your side, as opening up your torso is a sign of vulnerability and trust and will signal that you feel relaxed in the conversation.

Another thing to be aware of is eye contact. Make sure that you provide a good amount of eye contact, especially when the other person is talking, as it shows that you are listening and taking an active interest in what they are saying.

5. Be empathetic

Being empathetic doesn't mean agreeing with what someone says or not challenging them. It means understanding why they say the things they do and recognising that there are significant cultural, personal and psychological reasons why people might respond in a certain way.

Ultimately, one of the crucial things to remember when going into a conversation is that the person you are talking to is potentially going to base part of their judgement of veganism on that conversation. It is therefore important that we are rational and level-headed, as people will be quick to disregard veganism not because of the arguments but because of the way the person they were speaking to made them feel. Research has shown that our memories are often based on the emotions we felt at a certain moment rather than what we actually remember of events. For example, if you have an argument with a loved one, you might not remember what the person exactly said, but you will remember how they made you feel. So we should try to facilitate a conversation where we ask important questions and stimulate a product- ive conversation but in a such a way that the person we are speaking to doesn't leave feeling like they have been attacked or castigated.

AFTERWORD:
A VEGAN WORLD WOULD
BE BETTER FOR EVERYONE

I distinctly remember the first time I saw a live pig up close. It was during my first visit to a sanctuary for animals rescued from farms and slaughterhouses. I had just arrived, and I was walking through the entrance area when this pig suddenly walked up beside me. I put my hand out and touched them and was surprised to find that they had bristly hairs all over their body. I had always thought of pigs as being these smooth, pink animals and had only ever really seen their bodies after they'd had all their hair burned off in a slaughterhouse.

I crouched down and looked at their face. They had floppy ears with holes in them, and I watched as they began sniffing through their flat snout, trying to work out if I had any food on me. On realising that I didn't, they walked off to wherever it was they had decided they wanted to go, making a few grunts along the way. I stood there and watched as they left, and I remember thinking how oddly graceful they looked. The way their hooves and legs moved made it seem as though they were wearing high heels, with the front of each hoof being flatter and wider and the back being more of an elongated point. Much to my amusement, their legs crossed in front of one another with every step they took, almost as if they were on a catwalk.

I then noticed the stump where their tail should have been. Pigs' tails are normally depicted as curly, yet this pig had practically no tail at all. I already knew that pigs have their tails cut off in farms, but I'd never seen an animal in person who had suffered this kind of mutilation. I thought about all the piglets who had had their tails cut off in farms just so they could end up on my plate. If this pig hadn't been rescued, the same fate would have awaited them. Instead of walking about happily on the lookout for some food or a nice comfy area to snooze in, they wouldn't exist in any capacity at all. Every inch of their body would have either been rendered down, ground up or consumed by probably hundreds of different people who would have digested them and then flushed them into a sewer.

Sometimes I find myself in a situation where I am unable to formulate the words to express how profoundly disturbing what we do to animals really is. We take a living, conscious being and nonchalantly dominate them and treat them with such little regard that not even their screams and cries will stop us from exploiting them. This content and happy pig walking off in front of me had no idea how lucky they were. Their day consisted of going from eating to sleeping to getting belly rubs. For millions of other pigs, their day would have consisted of going from the farm onto a truck and then into a gas chamber.

I strongly believe that what we do to animals is something that future generations will look back at in horror. At the risk of sounding too idealistic, I hope that those future generations will be ones that come about in my lifetime. Although if they do, we should probably start to think about our answers to the questions, 'Why did you allow this to happen?

Why did you ever allow an industry that caused so much suffering, pain and death? That destroyed the natural world and the wildlife that existed within it, that caused infectious diseases, pandemics and antibiotic resistance, not to mention the chronic diseases and illnesses that affected hundreds of millions of people. What were you thinking?'

The truth is that we don't see the damage caused when we take a bite out of an animal product, but that doesn't make the damage any less real. Our ignorance about what is happening doesn't lessen the reality of what others are forced to endure as a consequence of our choices. I hope that this book has gone some way to revealing the enormity of the destruction and damage we cause to animals, but in reality I have only scratched the surface. I keep thinking that I've learned all there is to learn about what happens to animals and then something else reveals itself.

I hope this book has confirmed to you or convinced you that there has to be a better way. One of the things I find most exciting about veganism is the opportunity it presents to us to create a better world. Humans, for all our flaws, are also capable of achieving some truly remarkable things. I think the future of food will be filled with many examples of our capacity for innovation and creativity. In fact, we are already witnessing many of these things coming to fruition, both from a technological perspective and from a societal perspective as well.

Veganism will come about as a result of the traits in humans that we are most proud of – ingenuity, intellectual honesty, progressiveness and self-reflection – while rejecting many of the traits that are most damaging – stubbornness, wilful ignorance, violence, selfishness and apathy. We are already seeing this in action, and though getting accurate population statistics is challenging, a clear theme is being revealed by polling and surveys: veganism is growing.

WE ALREADY HAVE THE SOLUTION

While animal farmers are involved in doing many of the things that I have criticised throughout this book, I don't believe that veganism needs to come at their expense; on the contrary, they are a part of the solution to the problems that currently exist.

It is estimated that global farm subsidies equal more than $1 million per minute but with only 1 per cent of that being given to farmers to benefit the environment. On top of that, an estimated $12 trillion a year is spent on hidden costs to the environment and human health that occur as a consequence of our current food system.[1]

Unfortunately, as it stands, taxpayers' money is being used to the detriment of our planet and every living being who calls it home. But it doesn't have to be this way. We can use this money to help farmers transition into plant-based agriculture, providing them with the skills and equipment they need and supporting them as they make the change, shifting to more sustainable forms of crop farming in the process, such as regenerative plant farming and no-till agriculture. Many farmers feel trapped within the system, financially unable to leave and psychologically pressured to keep going because their farms have been passed on in their family from generation to generation. However, we can help ensure that the farmers who want to can stay in agriculture and keep producing food.

That said, because we don't want to turn all animal farms into arable farms, and many animal farms are on land that wouldn't be suitable anyway, we could also use the money to pay farmers to restore, reforest and rewild their farmland. In essence, they would be publicly funded land managers, subsidised by the state, but the commodity they would be providing wouldn't be food but instead wildflower meadows, forests, woodlands and peatlands. Rather than making a living from killing animals, they would be paid to provide habitats for wildlife and biodiversity – paid to create life, not to take it.

There is a precedent for this exact model of land stewardship. In the 1940s, around 75 per cent of Costa Rica was covered in rainforests. However, by the 1970s and 1980s, it had one of the highest rates of deforestation in Latin America, with as much as half of the forest cover being destroyed, primarily for cattle grazing and the production of animal feed. In response to this, the Costa Rican government made deforestation illegal, except for specifically approved reasons. They then introduced the Payments for Environmental Services Program, a subsidy system that paid farmers to protect biodiversity, sequester carbon-dioxide emissions and regrow the lost forests on the grazing lands.

Essentially, the government eliminated harmful payments such as cattle subsidies and replaced them with support payments for improving nature. As a result, Costa Rica has become the first tropical country to not only stop deforestation but actually reverse it as well. Around 60 per cent of land in Costa Rica is now covered by rainforests again, and they are home to hundreds of thousands of plant and animal species. The government raised money for the scheme through a tax on fossil fuels, which was then passed on to the farmers. One farmer, who replanted his farmland with trees through the scheme, said, 'I feel proud when I walk through the forest, not only for me but for my whole family . . . when I am no longer here, I know that my children will continue to look after it.'[2]

As it stands, an astonishing amount of money is squandered just keeping animal agriculture profitable. In the EU, 20 per cent (more than £24 billion) of the entire annual budget is spent subsidising animal farming.[3] In the UK, grazing animal farmers rely on subsidies for more than 90 per cent of their profits while only 10 per cent of the annual profits for fruit farmers comes from subsidy payments.[4] However, post-Brexit, there are changes being implemented to the UK's agriculture subsidies with the new Environmental Land Management Scheme awarding payments for environmental efforts such as improving soil health and restoring woodlands. But, with the transition to the new subsidy scheme lasting seven years, and many of the initiatives simply consisting of reversing some of the damage caused by a decade of deregulation by the same political party that is now attempting to incentivise the very measures it had previously been rallying against, it remains to be seen how impactful it will be.

In the USA, direct government aid to farmers rose to a record $46.5 billion in 2020, equalling about 40 per cent of net farm income. While we were being told that the pandemic was having a huge effect on farmers, these direct payments meant that US agriculture had its third most profitable year in half a century.[5] They were being increased at the same time that President Trump was trying to cut funding for food stamps, which would have seen 700,000 people lose access to them during the pandemic, neatly demonstrating where our current priorities lie.

These subsidies are being given to allow the practices that have been discussed in this book to continue. Through our taxes, we are in essence funding the animal cruelty, human exploitation, environmental degradation and disease creation that we should all want to bring to an end. Then, to add insult to injury, we are paying for the healthcare costs, the environmental clean-up costs and the pandemic costs that come about as a result of what we do to animals. It is a truly absurd, scandalous and immoral use of public funds – tax revenues are meant to be spent on improving society, not degrading and destroying it. We have the money; it just needs to be distributed in a fair and logical manner.

We should also tax animal products to reflect their true cost to society. Research has shown that there would need to be a 20 per cent tax on unprocessed meat and a 110 per cent tax on processed meat in high-income nations just to cover the healthcare costs incurred by the consumption of animal flesh.[6] Doing so would also cut annual deaths by 220,000 and save £130 billion a year. Another piece of research calculated that in the EU meat prices would have to rise by 40 per cent, organic meat prices would have to rise by 25 per cent and milk prices would have to rise by around 30 per cent to cover the environmental costs associated with their production.[7] In the same way that we have taxes on harmful products such as sugar, alcohol and tobacco, it makes logical and financial sense that the same be done for animal products. Why are we spending billions on these industries when doing so is causing hundreds of thousands of unnecessary deaths (hundreds of billions when you factor in the animals), and costing us even more money and destroying the environment? Let's reclaim this public money and redistribute it to help farmers, help animals, help the planet and help us. Then by taxing animal products so that consumers are paying the true cost of these products we can use the extra money generated to further implement positive strategies for a prosperous future.

THE SKY'S THE LIMIT

Just as in Costa Rica, the funds raised by recalibrating farm subsidies and a rethink of our taxation policies could be used in a similar way all around the world, with landowners also being able to generate income through agro-forestry and ecotourism. On top of that, jobs would be provided due to the maintenance that would be required on the land, meaning the people who have often found them-selves with little option other than to work in factory farms and slaughterhouses would instead be able to work in nature, thereby reducing stress, anxiety and mental health problems rather than creating them.[8]

In addition, to reduce the burden on our soils and increase food security, we can also use the money no longer being spent subsidising animal farming to create vertical farms. This is a method of agriculture that involves growing crops in ver-tically stacked layers. The farms are indoor units where the environment can be controlled, which means you can grow food all year round and the yield won't be affected by adverse weather conditions. One acre of vertical farm can produce the equivalent amount of food that would be grown on between 10 and 20 acres of a traditional soil-based farm.[9]

The plants are grown using a hydroponic system of re-cycled and filtered water, which means that less than 10 per cent of the amount of water is needed compared to trad-itional farming.[10] Not to mention that there's no need for pesticides and herbicides, no soil erosion, agricultural runoff or harmful methods of crop harvesting. And this system can be powered by renewable energy. You can produce food in the middle of cities and reduce the amount of travel miles and emissions. There are even facilities called deep farms, which are similar in concept but built in disused underground tunnels.

We have also begun to create meat without the slaughter-ing of any animals. Cultured meat is created by taking animal cells, mixing them with a liquid growth medium, which con-tains proteins, sugars and vitamins, and then placing them in a bioreactor – a machine that is often used to ferment beer.

Once in the bioreactor, the animal cells begin to grow and multiply until they start to look like meat. This meat can then be shaped to form foods such as burgers, nuggets and sausages, and companies are working on ways to create realistic cuts of meat, like steaks.

Cell-cultured meat removes the need to farm and kill an animal, and the product is actual meat. So not only does it have the potential to eliminate animal farming and all the suffering it inflicts on sentient beings, it can drastically reduce the environmental impact of meat production as well. Not only that, but it doesn't require the use of any antibiotics or hormones and wouldn't be contaminated with E. coli and other forms of bacteria that cause food poisoning, as well as removing the risk from bird flu, swine flu or any other infectious disease caused by the animal-farming industries. Because the production of cultured meat is created from the initial cells up, the nutrient levels can also be controlled, so you could theoretically reduce the fat and cholesterol and add more vitamins and healthy fats instead. It could be fortified in the same way we fortify breads and milk. Cell-cultured meat has already begun to be sold commercially, with the first product becoming publicly available in Singapore in late 2020.[11]

THE TIME FOR VEGANISM IS NOW

We have the capability to produce more food, in a healthier way, more sustainably and more ethically, while at the same time using less resources and land, producing fewer emissions, and eliminating the needless death of trillions of animals every single year. That number is so large that it can be difficult to grasp what it represents – individuals who are living their own subjective lives; individuals like the first pig I ever met, their chopped-off tail waggling just as much as it could as they walked away.

We all live by values given to us by the societies and cultures that we were raised in, reinforced by our parents and peers, and rationalised and defended by our cognitive biases. However, society has always progressed because we have challenged dominant paradigms and ingrained norms. The stagnation of progress comes from apathy, complacency and the refusal to critically reflect. We often look back through humanity's short history in disbelief at the way that we have acted in the past. Future generations will do the same when they reflect on the actions of our contemporary society unless we do the work that is required to shed our past transgressions. That work is still ongoing and in many regards is just beginning.

We currently treat the lives of others as being expendable and worthless. 'It's just a pig,' we might say. Or, 'They're only a chicken.' But to that pig and that chicken, their life is everything to them. Behind their eyes is a thinking, feeling individual. In the same way that each of us is not 'just a human' but instead a complex individual, our body simply a vessel through which we experience our life, the same is true of non-human animals. They may look different to us, talk differently to us, behave differently to us, but intrinsically they are not that dissimilar to us, especially not in the ways that matter morally. They are alive, they are conscious, they feel, they can suffer, they have families and friends, they seek comfort and safety.

One of the defining traits of our species is our ability to change, to learn from our mistakes and to evolve accordingly. Our morality has always changed, as has our understanding of the complexity and wonder of life itself. So is it not time to progress to the next step, to recognise that violence towards animals is not a rarity but instead systemic and ubiquitous, to acknowledge that we need to act now for the future of the planet and the potential survival of not just our own species but all species?

It's not an exaggeration to say that every single being in the world is negatively impacted by our consumption of animal products. Even those who earn their livings within the industry are affected by what is happening to our planet and the repercussions of animal farming. Everybody loses under the current system – but the flip side to that is that everybody wins when we change it.

Animal farming industries may like to believe that they are discrediting vegans by referring to the arguments in favour of veganism as 'propaganda' – in reality, they are instead attempting to discredit science, moral intuition and progress. Donald Watson, who coined the word vegan in 1944, once said, 'Veganism gives us all the opportunity to say what we stand for in life.' We have the power every day to either stand in favour of needless animal suffering, the destruction of our natural world and the increased risk of infectious disease and pandemics, or to stand against it. Which do we choose?

ACKNOWLEDGEMENTS

Reading has always been one of my favourite things to do. Growing up I read countless books and in doing so I amassed a large collection of Penguin Modern Classics with the spines displaying the Penguin logo pointing out from my bookshelf, inviting me to pick one of them up. When I looked at the spines I would envision one day having my own published book displaying the Penguin logo, so to Sam Jackson, thank you so much for for not only making my dream come true, but for also giving me the opportunity to write a book about veganism. I appreciate your trust and belief in me and I'm forever grateful to you for making this book a reality.

A huge thank you also to Marta, Jessica, Katie and everyone else in the Penguin Random House team for all of your work in bringing this book to life.

To Paul, it's been an absolute pleasure working with you. Thank you for helping me refine my ideas and for helping me express what I wanted to say in this book. Your observations and scrutiny of the arguments within this book have made it stronger and I am incredibly grateful to you for helping me throughout this project. The same is true for Liz, thank you for all of your hard work going through the book so meticulously.

A huge thank you to Josephine Hayes, without you this book wouldn't exist. I am so indebted to you for giving me the confidence to write a book and for reaching out to me in the first place with the purpose of encouraging me to write a book about veganism. Thank you to Rory and Hattie for pushing me to keep improving during those early stages and thank you to Grace for helping me find my voice in the initial proposal.

To my partner Luna, where would I be without you? Thank you for pushing me towards veganism in the first place and for being an instrumental part of this journey ever since. I would never have been given this opportunity if it wasn't for you and everything you do to support me and the work that we do together. Thank you for your patience and support whilst I spent day after day, week after week writing in the corner of our apartment.

To everyone who has supported my work throughout the years, thank you for everything. Thank you for giving my work a platform, thank you for supporting me and thank you for trusting in me. I really hope that you like this book.

To Rupert the Hamster, little did I know when I first saw you in a pet shop in Camden that you would have such a huge impact on my life. Thank you for helping me realise the hypocrisy of how I viewed different animals and for bringing joy to my life for the three years you were alive. I hope that you enjoyed your life with Luna and I. We loved you so much.

Finally, to all the animals who continue to suffer because of what we humans do, I am so deeply sorry. I hope that we one day look back in rightful dismay at what we currently force you to endure.

ENDNOTES

Introduction

1. http://www.fao.org/faostat/en/#data/QL
2. http://fishcount.org.uk/fish-count-estimates-2/numbers-of-fish-caught-from-the-wild-each-year

Chapter 1

1. Sato, N., Tan, L., Tate, K. *et al.* 'Rats demonstrate helping behavior toward a soaked conspecific', *Animal Cognition*, 18: 1039–47 (2015)
2. Reimert I., Bolhuis J. E., Kemp B., Rodenburg T. B. 'Emotions on the loose: emotional contagion and the role of oxytocin in pigs', *Animal Cognition*, 18, 517–32 (2015)
3. de Waal, F. B. M. 'Anthropomorphism and Anthropodenial: Consistency in Our Thinking about Humans and Other Animals', *Philosophical Topics*, 27, 1: 255–80 (1999), www.jstor.org/stable/43154308
4. de Waal, F. 'What I learned from tickling apes', *The New York Times,* 10 April 2016, https://www.nytimes.com/2016/04/10/opinion/sunday/what-i-learned-from-tickling-apes.html
5. Loughnan S., Bastian B., Haslam N. 'The Psychology of Eating Animals', *Current Directions in Psychological Science*, 23, 2: 104–8 (2014)
6. Ritchie, H. 'Cutting down forests: what are the drivers of deforestation?', *Our World in Data,* February 2021, https://ourworldindata.org/what-are-drivers-deforestation
7. Machovina, B. Feeley, K. J., Ripple, W. J. 'Biodiversity conservation: The key is reducing meat consumption', *Science of the Total Environment*, 536: 419–31 (2015)

Chapter 2

1. https://www.ers.usda.gov/data-products/ag-and-food-statistics-charting-the-essentials/farming-and-farm-income
2. https://www.sentienceinstitute.org/press/animal-farming-attitudes-survey-2017

3. Fellows, J. A. *et al.* 'The evolution and changing ecology of the African hominid oral microbiome', *Proceedings of the National Academy of Sciences*, 118, 20 (2021)
4. Harvard University, 'Turns out developing a taste for carbs wasn't a bad thing: Findings on Neanderthal oral microbiomes offer new clues on evolution, health', ScienceDaily, 10 May 2021, https://www.sciencedaily.com/releases/2021/05/210510161448.htm
5. Roser, M., Ritchie, H., and Ortiz-Ospina, E. 'World Population Growth', *Our World in Data*, May 2019, https://ourworldindata.org/world-population-growth
6. Atkins P.J., 'Mother's milk and infant death in Britain, circa 1900–1940', *Anthropology of Food* [Online], 2 September 2003, https://journals.openedition.org/aof/310
7. Lawrence, F., 'Rotten meat and bottled formaldehyde: fighting for food safety', *Nature* 562: 334–5 (2018)
8. Atkins, P. J. 'Sophistication detected: or, the adulteration of the milk supply, 1850–1914', *Social History*, 16, 3: 317–39 (1991)
9. Moodie, A. 'Fowl play: the chicken farmers being bullied by big poultry', *Guardian*, 22 April 2017, https://www.theguardian.com/sustainable-business/2017/apr/22/chicken-farmers-big-poultry-rules
10. Wasley, A. *et al.* 'JBS: The Brazilian butchers who took over the world', *The Bureau of Investigative Journalism*, 2 July 2019, https://www.thebureauinvestigates.com/stories/2019-07-02/jbs-brazilian-butchers-took-over-the-world
11. Wasley, A. and Kroker, H. 'Revealed: Industrial-scale beef farming comes to the UK', *Guardian*, 29 May 2018, https://www.theguardian.com/environment/2018/may/29/revealed-industrial-scale-beef-farming-comes-to-the-uk

Chapter 3

1. https://api.worldanimalprotection.org
2. Webster, B. 'Red Tractor accepts need for change as shoppers want more spot checks', *The Times*, 30 July 2018, https://www.thetimes.co.uk/article/farm-animals-tortured-under-red-tractor-label-rcbrhxqlm
3. Dalton, J. 'Farm banned by Red Tractor for pig cruelty supplies meat to major wholesalers', *Independent*, 15 June 2020, https://www.independent.co.uk/climate-change/news/pig-animal-cruelty-red-tractor-rosebury-farm-dunstable-inspectors-ban-a8470011.html
4. Poulter, S. 'Tesco suspends sales of chicken from an "ethical" farm after an undercover probe by animal rights activists revealed shocking abuse of the birds', *Daily Mail*, 30 June 2019, https://www.

dailymail.co.uk/news/article-7198811/Tesco-suspends-sales-chicken-ethical-farm-undercover-probe-reveals-shocking-abuse.html

5. https://animalequality.org/news/investigation-suffering-abuse-and-cannibalism-filmed-on-british-chicken-farms

6. Dalton, J. 'Farm banned by Red Tractor for pig cruelty'

7. Mellor D. J. 'Updating Animal Welfare Thinking: Moving beyond the "Five Freedoms" towards "A Life Worth Living"', *Animals*, 6(3), 21, (2016)

8. https://www.rspcaassured.org.uk/about-us/farm-assessments

9. https://www.rspcaassured.org.uk/about-us/rspca-monitoring

10. Macaskill, M. 'RSPCA paid over £500,000 to back Scottish salmon industry', *The Times*, 9 February 2020, https://www.thetimes.co.uk/article/rspca-paid-over-500-000-to-back-scottish-salmon-industry-bqcn7gs22

11. Compassion in World Farming, 'Murky depths of the Scottish salmon industry exposed in new undercover investigation', 23 March 2021, https://www.ciwf.org.uk/news/2021/03/murky-depths-of-the-scottish-salmon-industry-exposed-in-new-undercover-investigation

12. Monbiot, G. 'The RSPCA rescues one seal – and condones the killing of many others', *Guardian*, 19 September 2018, https://www.theguardian.com/commentisfree/2018/sep/19/rspca-seal-charity-fish-farms-seals

13. Carrell, S. 'Scottish salmon farmers to be banned from shooting seals', *Guardian*, 17 June 2020, https://www.theguardian.com/world/2020/jun/17/scottish-salmon-farmers-to-be-banned-from-shooting-seals

14. Rivera, L. 'Unmasking the truth behind food labelling in the chicken industry', *Independent*, 4 June 2017, https://www.independent.co.uk/life-style/food-and-drink/supermarket-chicken-labels-truth-free-range-battery-treatment-organic-a7751536.html

15. https://www.rspca.org.uk/whatwedo/howwework/policies/vegetarianism

16. https://www.rspca.org.uk/-/9429126

17. https://www.gov.uk/guidance/farm-animals-looking-after-their-welfare

18. Wasley, A., Robbins, J. 'Severe welfare breaches recorded six times a day in British slaughterhouses', *The Bureau of Investigative Journalism*, 28 August 2016, https://www.thebureauinvestigates.com/stories/2016-08-28/severe-welfare-breaches-recorded-six-times-a-day-in-british-slaughterhouses

19. Morrison, O. ' "How much more likely do you think you would be to make a mistake if someone was stood watching over you?" Lawyer takes aim at "zero-tolerance" abattoir rules', *Food Navigator*, 10 December 2020, https://www.foodnavigator.com/Article/2020/12/10/Lawyer-takes-aim-at-zero-tolerance-abattoir-rules

20. Animal Aid, 'Britain's failing slaughterhouses: why it's time to make independently monitored CCTV mandatory', 2017, https://www.animalaid.org.uk/wp-content/uploads/2017/05/Britains-Failing-Slaughterhouses-v6.pdf

21. https://faunalytics.org/global-pig-slaughter-statistics-and-charts

22. Mutimer, R. 'Opinion: More challenges ahead for hard-pressed pig farmers', *Eastern Daily Press*, 4 May 2021, https://www.edp24.co.uk/news/business/npa-chairman-rob-mutimer-on-pig-farming-challenges-7933680

23. Ceballos, M. C., Rocha Góis, K. C., Parsons, T. D., Pierdon, M. 'Impact of Duration of Farrowing Crate Closure on Physical Indicators of Sow Welfare and Piglet Mortality', *Animals*, 11, 4: 969 (2021).

24. Mutimer, R. 'Opinion: More challenges ahead'

25. Rivera, Lizzie. The truth behind the pork we eat, *The Independent*, June 2017. https://www.independent.co.uk/life-style/food-and-drink/pork-production-truth-pig-farming-uk-factory-hughfearnley-whittingstall-sienna-miller-mick-jagger-a7813746.html

26. https://www.rspca.org.uk/adviceandwelfare/farm/pigs/farming

27. Rivera, L. 'The truth behind the pork we eat', *Independent*, 29 June 2017, https://www.independent.co.uk/life-style/food-and-drink/pork-production-truth-pig-farming-uk-factory-hughfearnley-whittingstall-sienna-miller-mick-jagger-a7813746.html

28. Farm Animal Welfare Committee, 'FAWC: Opinion on the welfare of animals killed on-farm', 29 March 2018, https://assets.publishing.service.gov.uk/government/uploads/system/uploads/attachment_data/file/695225/fawc-opinion-welfare-of-animals-killed-on-farm-march2018.pdf

29. https://viva.org.uk/animals/campaigns/pigs/investigation-flat-house-farm

30. https://animalequality.org.uk/news/pigs-hammered-to-death-on-high-welfare-farm

31. National Pig Association, 'NPA responds to consumer concerns over method of dispatching sick piglets', 1 August 2018. http://www.npa-uk.org.uk/NPA_responds_to_consumer_concerns_over_method_of_dispatching_sick_piglets.html

32. Çavuşoğlu E., *et al*. 'Behavioral Response of Weaned Pigs during Gas Euthanasia with CO2, CO2 with Butorphanol, or Nitrous Oxide', *Animals*, 10, 5: 787 (2020)

33. Verhoeven M., *et al*. 'Time to Loss of Consciousness and Its Relation to Behavior in Slaughter Pigs during Stunning with 80 or 95% Carbon Dioxide'. *Frontiers in Veterinary Science* 3, 38 (2016)

34. Farm Animal Welfare Committee, 'Report on the Welfare of Farmed Animals at Slaughter or Killing. Part 1: Red Meat Animals', June 2003,

https://assets.publishing.service.gov.uk/government/uploads/system/
uploads/attachment_data/file/325241/FAWC_report_on_the_
welfare_of_farmed_animals_at_slaughter_or_killing_part_one_red_
meat_animals.pdf

35. DEFRA, 'Results of the 2018 FSA Survey into Slaughter Methods
in England and Wales', February 2019, https://assets.publishing.
service.gov.uk/government/uploads/system/uploads/attachment_
data/file/778588/slaughter-method-survey-2018.pdf

36. Agriculture Bill, Written evidence submitted by Compassion in
World Farming, February 2020, https://publications.parliament.
uk/pa/cm5801/cmpublic/Agriculture/memo/AB03.htm

37. Robbins J. A., et al. 'Factors influencing public support for dairy tie
stall housing in the U.S.', PLoS ONE, 14, 5 (2019)

38. Ibid.

39. Levitt, T. ' "It's medieval": why some cows are still living most of
their lives tied up', Guardian, 8 December 2018, https://www.
theguardian.com/environment/2018/dec/08/its-medieval-why-
some-cows-are-still-living-most-of-their-lives-tied-up

40. https://www.nfuonline.com/great-british-beef-week-sucklers-2

41. EFSA AHAW Panel (EFSA Panel on Animal Health and Animal
Welfare), More, S, et al. 'Scientific Opinion on the animal welfare
aspects in respect of the slaughter or killing of pregnant livestock
animals (cattle, pigs, sheep, goats, horses)', EFSA Journal, 15, 5:
4782, 96 pp. (2017)

42. RSPCA, RSPCA welfare standards for dairy cattle, January 2018,
https://science.rspca.org.uk/documents/1494935/9042554/RSPCA+
welfare+standards+for+dairy+cattle+%28PDF+7.76MB%29.pdf/
41638530-20de-c6cc-5e9c-7b73f9c8f4b7?t=1557731468543

43. Mann, T. 'Shocking pictures show young cows crammed into cages at
M&S dairy farm', Metro, 3 March 2017, https://metro.
co.uk/2017/03/28/shocking-pictures-show-young-cows-crammed-
into-cages-at-ms-dairy-farm-6538507

44. https://www.ciwf.org.uk/farm-animals/cows/veal-calves

45. Dalton, J. 'Morrisons aims to halt practice of shooting male calves
at birth', Independent, 21 August 2019, https://www.independent.
co.uk/climate-change/news/morrisons-meat-male-calves-dairy-
shot-birth-farms-a9073821.html

46. https://expiredcampaign.org/dairystillkills

47. Wasley, A., Kroeker, H. 'Revealed: industrial-scale beef farming
comes to the UK', The Bureau of Investigative Journalism, 29 May
2018, https://www.thebureauinvestigates.com/stories/2018-05-29/
inside-britains-new-intensive-agriculture-sector-beef-lots

48. Southworth, P. 'Cattle farmers campaign to lower age cows can be
killed and sold as beef', Telegraph, 13 September 2019, https://

www.telegraph.co.uk/news/2019/09/13/cattle-farmers-campaign-lower-age-cows-can-killed-sold-beef

49. Atkinson, S., Velarde, A., Algers, B. 'Assessment of stun quality at commercial slaughter in cattle shot with captive bolt', *Animal Welfare*, 22 (2013)

50. https://ec.europa.eu/food/sites/food/files/animals/docs/aw_prac_slaughter_factsheet-2018_stun_cattle_en.pdf

51. Warrick, J. 'They die piece by piece', *Washington Post*, 10 April 2001, https://www.washingtonpost.com/archive/politics/2001/04/10/they-die-piece-by-piece/f172dd3c-0383-49f8-b6d8-347e04b68da1

52. *Ibid.*

53. Elder, M. 'Why your chicken wings mean we've entered a new epoch', *Guardian*, 10 January 2019, https://www.theguardian.com/commentisfree/2019/jan/10/chicken-modern-factory-farm-anthropocene-new-age

54. Rivera, L. 'Unmasking the truth behind food labelling in the chicken industry', *Independent*, 4 June 2017, https://www.independent.co.uk/life-style/food-and-drink/supermarket-chicken-labels-truth-free-range-battery-treatment-organic-a7751536.html

55. https://www.sentienceinstitute.org/us-factory-farming-estimates

56. Caffyn, A. 'Revealed: true cost of Britain's addiction to factory-farmed chicken', *The Conversation*, 19 April 2021, https://theconversation.com/revealed-true-cost-of-britains-addiction-to-factory-farmed-chicken-158555

57. https://www.rspca.org.uk/adviceandwelfare/farm/meatchickens/farming

58. Lawrence, F. 'If consumers knew how farmed chickens were raised, they might never eat their meat again', *Guardian*, 24 April 2016, https://www.theguardian.com/environment/2016/apr/24/real-cost-of-roast-chicken-animal-welfare-farms

59. Schwean-Lardner, K., Classen, Dr H. 'Lighting for Broilers', *Aviagen*, 2010. https://eu.aviagen.com/assets/Tech_Center/Broiler_Breeder_Tech_Articles/English/LightingforBroilers1.pdf

60. Aziz, Dr T., Barnes, Dr H. J. 'Harmful effects of ammonia on birds', *Poultry World*, 25 October 2010, https://www.poultryworld.net/Breeders/Health/2010/10/Harmful-effects-of-ammonia-on-birds-WP008071W

61. Colley, C., Wasley, A. 'Over 60 million chickens in England and Wales rejected over disease and defects', *Guardian*, 25 August 2020, https://www.theguardian.com/environment/2020/aug/25/over-60-million-chickens-in-england-and-wales-rejected-over-disease-and-defects

62. Webster, B. 'A million chickens die on way to abattoirs as violations rise', *The Times*, 7 September 2018, https://www.thetimes.co.uk/article/a-million-chickens-die-on-way-to-abattoirs-as-violations-rise-208p8b5nj

63. Berg C., Raj M. 'A Review of Different Stunning Methods for Poultry-Animal Welfare Aspects (Stunning Methods for Poultry)', *Animals*, 5, 4: 1207–19 (2015)

64. Nicholson, R. 'What does "free-range" actually mean? It's complicated', *Guardian*, 28 February 2017, https://www.theguardian.com/lifeandstyle/shortcuts/2017/feb/28/what-does-free-range-actually-mean-its-complicated

65. https://www.egginfo.co.uk/egg-facts-and-figures/industry-information/data

66. https://www.ciwf.com/media/7442448/2020-eggtrack-report-english.pdf

67. DEFRA, 'Code of practice for the welfare of laying hens and pullets', 2018, https://assets.publishing.service.gov.uk/government/uploads/system/uploads/attachment_data/file/732227/code-of-practice-welfare-of-laying-hens-pullets.pdf

68. Farm Animal Welfare Council, 'Opinion on osteoporosis and bone fractures in laying hens', December 2010, https://edepot.wur.nl/161696

69. *Ibid.*

70. http://adlib.everysite.co.uk/resources/000/107/984/lambsurvival.pdf

71. http://www.fao.org/faostat/en/#data/QL

72. http://fishcount.org.uk/fish-count-estimates-2/numbers-of-fish-caught-from-the-wild-each-year

73. Diarte-Plata, G. *et al.* 'Eyestalk ablation procedures to minimize pain in the freshwater prawn Macrobrachium americanum', *Applied Animal Behaviour Science*, 140: 172–8 (2012)

74. 'Scientific opinion of the panel on Animal Health and Welfare on a request from European Commission on general approach to fish welfare and to the concept of sentience in fish', *EFSA Journal* 954: 1–26 (2009) https://efsa.onlinelibrary.wiley.com/doi/pdf/10.2903/j.efsa.2009.954

75. Robb, D., Kestin, S. C. 'Methods Used to Kill Fish: Field Observations and Literature Reviewed', *Animal Welfare* 11: 269–82 (2002)

76. Nilsson, J. *et al.* 'Sudden exposure to warm water causes instant behavioural responses indicative of nociception or pain in Atlantic salmon', *Veterinary and Animal Science* 8: 10007 (2019)

77. https://donstaniford.typepad.com/files/thermolicer-foi-18-01466---mortality-event-reports---june-2018.pdf

78. Mann, J. 'Millions of dead salmon dumped, burnt, or destroyed by Scottish salmon farms', *The National*, 21 March 2021, https://www.thenational.scot/news/19175990.millions-dead-salmon-dumped-burnt-destroyed-scottish-salmon-farms

79. https://viva.org.uk/animals/campaigns/investigation-rainbow-trout

80. McDonald, G. G. *et al.* 'Satellites can reveal global extent of forced labor in the world's fishing fleet', *Proceedings of the National Academy of Sciences* 118, 3 (2021)

81. Mason, M. *et al.* 'Shrimp sold by global supermarkets is peeled by slave labourers in Thailand', *Guardian,* 14 December 2015, https://www.theguardian.com/global-development/2015/dec/14/shrimp-sold-by-global-supermarkets-is-peeled-by-slave-labourers-in-thailand

82. Floor Borlée, C., *et al.* 'Air Pollution from Livestock Farms Is Associated with Airway Obstruction in Neighboring Residents', *American Journal of Respiratory and Critical Care Medicine* 196, 9 (2017)

83. Domingo, N. G. G. *et al.* 'Air quality-related health damages of food', *Proceedings of the National Academy of Sciences* 118, 20 (2021)

84. Human Rights Watch, 'Toxic tanneries: the health repercussions of Bangladesh's Hazaribagh leather', 8 October 2012, https://www.hrw.org/report/2012/10/08/toxic-tanneries/health-repercussions-bangladeshs-hazaribagh-leather

85. Srivastava, R. 'Indian leather workers risk health, life to make shoes for global market: report', *Reuters,* 15 March 2017, https://www.reuters.com/article/indian-leather-workers-risk-health-life-idUSL5N1GS5U3

86. Rastogi S. K., *et al.* 'Occupational cancers in leather tanning industries: A short review', *Indian Journal of Occupational and Environmental Medicine* 11, 1: 3–5 (2007)

87. Equality and Human Rights Commission, 'Inquiry into recruitment and employment in the meat and poultry processing sector. Coercion, physical and verbal abuse of agency workers: our findings.' 2010

88. Wasley, A.. 'Revealed: shocking safety record of UK meat plants', *The Bureau of Investigative Journalism,* 20 April 2017. https://www.thebureauinvestigates.com/stories/2017-04-20/bullying-harassment-and-physical-assault-abuse-faced-by-inspectors-inside-uk-slaughterhouses

89. Wasley, A., Heal, A. 'Revealed: shocking safety record of UK meat plants', *The Bureau of Investigative Journalism,* 29 July 2018, https://www.thebureauinvestigates.com/stories/2018-07-29/uk-meat-plant-injuries

90. Hutz, C., Zanon, C., Neto, H. 'Adverse Working Conditions and Mental Illness in Poultry Slaughterhouses in Southern Brazil', *Psicologia: Reflexão e Crítica* 26: 296–304 (2012)

91. https://www.oxfamamerica.org/livesontheline

92. 'Slaughterhouse worker opens up: "It was a vision of Hell" ', *Plant Based News,* 20 October 2017, https://plantbasednews.org/opinion/plantbased-vegan-slaughterhouse-abattoir-hell

Chapter 4

1. Steinfeld, H. 'Livestock's Long Shadow: Environmental Issues and Options', UN report, Food and Agriculture Organization of the United Nations, 2006

2. Carus, F. 'UN urges global move to meat and dairy-free diet', *Guardian,* 2 June 2010, https://www.theguardian.com/environment/2010/jun/02/un-report-meat-free-diet

3. Harwatt, H., Hayek, M. N. 'Eating away at climate change with negative emissions: repurposing UK agricultural land to meet climate goals', *Harvard Law School,* April 2019

4. Monbiot, G. 'Explanation of the figures in grim reaping', 11 January 2017,https://www.monbiot.com/2017/01/11/explanation-of-the-figures-in-grim-reaping

5. Merrill, D., Leatherby, L. 'Here's how America uses its land', *Bloomberg,* 31 July 2018, https://www.bloomberg.com/graphics/2018-us-land-use

6. Searchinger, T., *et al.* 'Creating a sustainable food future: A menu of solutions to feed nearly 10 billion people by 2050', *World Resources Institute,* December 2018.

7. Steinfeld, H. 'Livestock's Long Shadow'.

8. Malm, L. *et al.* 'Livestock grazing impacts components of the breeding productivity of a common upland insectivorous passerine: Results from a long-term experiment.' *Journal of Applied Ecology* 57 (2020)

9. Hayhow, D. B. *et al.* 'State of Nature 2016', The State of Nature partnership (2016)

10. Poore, J., Nemecek, T. 'Reducing food's environmental impacts through producers and consumers', *Science*, 1 June 2018

11. Carrington, D. 'UK's native woodlands reaching crisis point, report warns', *Guardian*, 14 April 2021, https://www.theguardian.com/environment/2021/apr/14/trees-uk-native-woodlands-reaching-crisis-point

12. Reid, C., *et al.* 'State of the UK's Woods and Trees 2021', Woodland Trust (2021)

13. Poore, J., Nemecek, T. 'Reducing food's environmental impacts'.

14. Shepon, A. *et al.* 'The opportunity cost of animal based diets exceeds all food losses', *Proceedings of the National Academy of Sciences of the United States of America* 115: 3804–9 (2018)

15. Harwatt, H., Hayek, M. N. 'Eating away at climate change with negative emissions'.

16. Sejian V. *et al.* 'Global Warming: Role of Livestock', in *Climate Change Impact on Livestock: Adaptation and Mitigation* (Springer, 2015)

17. IPCC, '2014: Climate Change 2014: Mitigation of Climate Change', contribution of Working Group III to the Fifth Assessment Report of the Intergovernmental Panel on Climate Change (Cambridge University Press, 2014)

18. Wolf, J., Asrar, G.R., West, T.O. 'Revised methane emissions factors and spatially distributed annual carbon fluxes for global livestock', *Carbon Balance Manage* 12, 16 (2017), https://doi.org/10.1186/s13021-017-0084-y

19. IPCC, '2021: Climate Change 2021: The Physical Science Basis. Contribution of Working Group I to the Sixth Assessment Report of the Intergovernmental Panel on Climate Change' (Cambridge University Press, 2021)

20. Volcovici, V. 'To save the planet, focus on cutting methane', UN climate report, R*euters,* 9 August 2021, https://www.reuters.com/business/environment/save-planet-focus-cutting-methane-un-climate-report-2021-08-09/

21. Poore J., Nemecek T. 'Reducing food's environmental impacts through producers and consumers', *Science* 360, 6392: 987–92 (2018)

22. *Ibid.*

23. Theurl, M.C. *et al.* 'Food systems in a zero-deforestation world: Dietary change is more important than intensification for climate targets in 2050', *Science of The Total Environment* 735, 139353 (2020)

24. Pieper, M., Michalke, A., Gaugler, T. 'Calculation of external climate costs for food highlights inadequate pricing of animal products', *Nature Communications* 11, 6117 (2020)

25. Poore J., Nemecek T., 'Reducing food's environmental impacts through producers and consumers'.

26. Sandström, V. *et al.* 'The role of trade in the greenhouse gas footprints of EU diets', *Global Food Security* 19: 48–55 (2018)

27. Weber, C. L., Scott Matthews, H., 'Food-Miles and the Relative Climate Impacts of Food Choices in the United States', *Environmental Science & Technology* 42, 10: 3508–13 (2008)

28. Carlsson-Kanyama, A., Pipping Ekström, M., Shanahan, H. 'Food and life cycle energy inputs: consequences of diet and ways to increase efficiency', *Ecological Economics* 44, 2–3: 293–307 (2003)

29. Ritchie, H. 'Very little of global food is transported by air; this greatly reduces the climate benefits of eating local', *Our World in Data,* 28 January 2020, https://ourworldindata.org/food-transport-by-mode

30. Ritchie, Hannah. 'Climate change and flying: what share of global CO2 emissions come from aviation?' *Our World in Data,* October 2020. https://ourworldindata.org/co2-emissions-from-aviation

31. Poore J., Nemecek T. 'Reducing food's environmental impacts through producers and consumers'.

32. Clark, M. *et al*. 'Global food system emissions could preclude achieving the 1.5° and 2°C climate change targets', *Science* 370, 6517: 705–8 (2020)

33. Springmann, M., *et al*. 'Options for keeping the food system within environmental limits', *Nature* 562: 519–25 (2018)

34. Benton, T. G. *et al*. 'Food system impacts on biodiversity loss: Three levers for food system transformation in support of nature', (Chatham House, 2021) https://www.chathamhouse.org/2021/02/food-system-impacts-biodiversity-loss

35. Garnett, T., *et al*. 'Grazed and Confused? Ruminating on cattle, grazing systems, methane, nitrous oxide, the soil carbon sequestration question – and what it all means for greenhouse gas emissions', (University of Oxford, 2014)

36. https://www.drawdown.org/solutions

37. Ceballos, G., Ehrlich, P., Dirzo, R. 'Biological annihilation via the ongoing sixth mass extinction signaled by vertebrate population losses and declines', Proceedings of the National Academy of Sciences 114 (2017)

38. Machovina, B., Feeley, K. J., Ripple, W. J. 'Biodiversity conservation: The key is reducing meat consumption', *Science of the Total Environment* 536: 419–31 (2015)

39. Bar-On, Y. M., Phillips, R., Milo, R. 'The biomass distribution on Earth', Proceedings of the National Academy of Sciences 115 (2018)

40. Bennett C. E. *et al*. 'The broiler chicken as a signal of a human reconfigured biosphere', *Royal Society Open Science* 5, 12 (2018)

41. Thomson, D. M., 'Local bumble bee decline linked to recovery of honey bees, drought effects on floral resources', *Ecology Letters* 19: 1247–55 (2016)

42. Garibaldi, L. *et al*. 'Wild Pollinators Enhance Fruit Set of Crops Regardless of Honey Bee Abundance', *Science* 339, 6127 (2013)

43. Valido, A., Rodríguez-Rodríguez, M. C., Jordano, P. 'Impact of the introduction of the domestic bee (Apis mellifera, Apidae) in the Teide National Park (Tenerife, Canary Islands)', *Ecosystems* 23, 3: 58–66 (2014)

44. University of Cambridge, 'Think of honeybees as "livestock" not wildlife, argue experts', 25 January 2018, https://www.cam.ac.uk/research/news/think-of-honeybees-as-livestock-not-wildlife-argue-experts

45. Turner, A. ' "Honeybees are voracious": is it time to put the brakes on the boom in beekeeping?', *Guardian*, 24 July 2021, https://www.theguardian.com/environment/2021/jul/24/this-only-saves-honeybees-the-trouble-with-britains-beekeeping-boom-aoe

46. https://www.theccc.org.uk/wp-content/uploads/2019/04/NFU-response-to-Call-for-Evidence-2018-1.pdf
47. https://www.desmog.com/agribusiness-database-agriculture-horticulture-development-board
48. https://assets.publishing.service.gov.uk/government/uploads/system/uploads/attachment_data/file/862887/2018_Final_green house_gas_emissions_statistical_release.pdf
49. https://assets.publishing.service.gov.uk/government/uploads/system/uploads/attachment_data/file/945470/ghgindicator-6dairycow-18dec20.pdf
50. Cobirka, M., Tancin, V., Slama, P. 'Epidemiology and Classification of Mastitis', *Animals* 10, 12: 2212 (2020)
51. Dworecka-Kaszak, B. *et al.* 'High prevalence of Candida yeast in milk samples from cows suffering from mastitis in Poland', *The Scientific World Journal* (2012)
52. https://www.gov.scot/publications/assessment-opportunities-retain-increase-sheep-lamb-processing-scotland/pages/3/#f-4
53. https://www.epicscotland.org/media/1118/epic-sheep-scenario-planning-report-final.pdf
54. https://www.gov.uk/government/statistics/food-statistics-pocketbook/food-statistics-in-your-pocket-global-and-uk-supply
55. https://assets.publishing.service.gov.uk/government/uploads/system/uploads/attachment_data/file/862887/2018_Final_green house_gas_emissions_statistical_release.pdf
56. https://www.efeca.com/wp-content/uploads/2019/12/UK-RT-on-Sustainable-Soya-APR-2019-final.pdf
57. https://www.efeca.com/wp-content/uploads/2019/12/UK-RT-on-Sustainable-Soya-APR-2019-final.pdf
58. https://resourcetrade.earth
59. Greenpeace, 'Winging it: How the UK's chicken habit is fuelling the climate and nature emergency', January 2020, https://www.greenpeace.org.uk/wp-content/uploads/2020/01/Greenpeace_WingingIt.pdf
60. Fraanje, W. 'Soy in the UK: What are its uses?', Table Debates, 20 February 2020, https://www.tabledebates.org/blog/soy-uk-what-are-its-uses
61. *Ibid.*
62. Fraanje, W., Garnett, T. 'Soy: food, feed, and land use change', Table Debates, 30 January 2020, https://www.tabledebates.org/building-blocks/soy-food-feed-and-land-use-change
63. https://www.gov.uk/government/statistics/food-statistics-pocket book/food-statistics-in-your-pocket-global-and-uk-supply
64. Fraanje, W., Garnett, T. 'Soy: food, feed, and land use change'.
65. *Ibid.*

66. https://wwf.panda.org/discover/our_focus/food_practice/sustainable_production/soy
67. Ortolani, G. 'Brazilian hunger for meat fattened on soy is deforesting the Cerrado: report', *Mongabay*, 16 January 2019, https://news.mongabay.com/2019/01/brazilian-hunger-for-meat-fattened-on-soy-is-deforesting-the-cerrado-report
68. Ritchie, H., Roser, M. 'Environmental impacts of food production', *Our World in Data*, June 2021, https://ourworldindata.org/environmental-impacts-of-food
69. https://www.food.gov.uk/business-guidance/gm-in-animal-feed
70. https://www.nfuonline.com/going-against-the-grain-report
71. de Ruiter, H. *et al.* 'Global cropland and greenhouse gas impacts of UK food supply are increasingly located overseas', *Journal of the Royal Society Interface* 13, 114 (2016)
72. https://assets.publishing.service.gov.uk/government/uploads/system/uploads/attachment_data/file/805926/State_of_the_environment_soil_report.pdf
73. Watts, J. 'Third of Earth's soil is acutely degraded due to agriculture', *Guardian*, 12 September 2017, https://www.theguardian.com/environment/2017/sep/12/third-of-earths-soil-acutely-degraded-due-to-agriculture-study
74. Poore, J., Nemecek, T., 'Reducing food's environmental impacts through producers and consumers', *Science* 360, 6392: 987–992 (2018)
75. *Ibid.*
76. https://www.nationalgeographic.org/encyclopedia/dead-zone
77. Mighty Earth, 'Mystery Meat II: The Industry Behind the Quiet Destruction of the American Heartland', 2017, http://www.mightyearth.org/wp-content/uploads/2017/08/Meat-Pollution-in-America.pdf
78. *Ibid.*
79. *Ibid.*
80. *Ibid.*
81. Tietz, J. 'Boss Hog: The Dark Side of America's Top Pork Producer', *Rolling Stone*, December 2006, https://www.rollingstone.com/culture/culture-news/boss-hog-the-dark-side-of-americas-top-pork-producer-68087
82. https://www.eea.europa.eu/themes/water/europes-seas-and-coasts/assessments/state-of-bathing-water/state-of-bathing-waters-in-2020
83. Laville, S. 'Shocking state of English rivers revealed as all of them fail pollution tests', *Guardian*, 17 September 2020, https://www.theguardian.com/environment/2020/sep/17/rivers-in-england-fail-pollution-tests-due-to-sewage-and-chemicals

84. Crisp, W. 'Revealed: no penalties issued under "useless" English farm pollution laws', *Guardian*, 12 February 2021, https://www.the-guardian.com/environment/2021/feb/12/revealed-no-penalties-issued-under-useless-uk-farm-pollution-laws

85. Monbiot, G. 'Think dairy farming is benign? Our rivers tell a different story', *Guardian*, 5 October 2015, https://www.theguardian.com/environment/2015/oct/05/think-dairy-farming-is-benign-our-rivers-tell-a-different-story

86. Monbiot, G. 'The government is looking the other way while Britain's rivers die before our eyes', *Guardian*, 12 August 2020, https://www.theguardian.com/commentisfree/2020/aug/12/government-britains-rivers-uk-waterways-farming-water-companies

87. https://salmon-trout.org/wp-content/uploads/2020/03/Final-Axe-Regulatory-Report.pdf

88. https://www.gov.uk/government/news/environment-secretary-calls-for-fewer-inspections-to-make-cap-simpler-for-farmers

89. https://www.gov.uk/government/speeches/environment-secretary-speech-at-the-oxford-farming-conference

90. Crisp, W. 'Revealed: no penalties issued under "useless" English farm pollution laws', *Guardian*, 12 February 2021, https://www.theguardian.com/environment/2021/feb/12/revealed-no-penalties-issued-under-useless-uk-farm-pollution-laws

91. Eveleigh, R. 'Welsh council admits it should not have approved vast poultry farm', *Guardian*, 30 January 2021, https://www.theguardian.com/environment/2021/jan/30/welsh-council-admits-it-should-not-have-approved-vast-poultry-farm

92. Gerbens-Leenes, W., Mekonnen, M., Hoekstra, A. 'The water footprint of poultry, pork and beef: A comparative study in different countries and production systems', *Water Resources and Industry* 1–2: 25–36 (2013)

93. Mekonnen, M., Hoekstra, A. 'The green, blue and grey water footprint of farm animals and animal products', (Unesco-IHE Institute for Water Education, 2010).

94. *Ibid.*

95. https://www.nationalgeographic.org/encyclopedia/dead-zone

96. *Ibid.*

97. https://oceanservice.noaa.gov/facts/ocean-oxygen.html

98. https://www.un.org/en/conferences/ocean2020/about

99. Chami, R. *et al.* 'Nature's Solution to climate change: A strategy to protect whales can limit greenhouse gases and global warming' (IMF, 2019), https://www.imf.org/external/pubs/ft/fandd/2019/12/pdf/natures-solution-to-climate-change-chami.pdf

100. https://oceanservice.noaa.gov/facts/oceanwater.html

101. Sala, E. *et al.* 'Protecting the global ocean for biodiversity, food and climate', *Nature* 592: 397–402 (2021)

102. Pershing, A. *et al.* 'The Impact of Whaling on the Ocean Carbon Cycle: Why Bigger Was Better', *PloS One* 5 (2010).
103. *Ibid.*
104. Chami, R. *et al.* 'Nature's Solution to climate change: A strategy to protect whales can limit greenhouse gases and global warming'
105. Roberts, C. *The Ocean of Life: The Fate of Man and the Sea* (Penguin Books, 2013)
106. Keledjian, A. 'Wasted catch: unsolved problems in U.S. fisheries' (Oceana, 2014), https://oceana.org/sites/default/files/Bycatch_Report_FINAL.pdf
107. *Ibid.*
108. Zeller, D. *et al.* 'Global marine fisheries discards: A synthesis of reconstructed data', *Fish Fish* 19: 30–9 (2018)
109. Neslen, A. 'Global fish production approaching sustainable limit, UN warns.' *Guardian,* 7 July 2016, https://www.theguardian.com/environ ment/2016/jul/07/global-fish-production-approaching-sustainable-limit-un-warns
110. Compassion in World Farming, 'Until the Seas Run Dry: How industrial aquaculture is plundering the oceans', April 2019. https://www.ciwf.org.uk/media/7436121/ex-summary-until-the-seas-dry.pdf
111. Thomas, K., Dorey, C., Obaidullah, F., 'Ghost gear: The abandoned fishing nets haunting our oceans', (Greenpeace Germany, 2019)
112. *Ibid.*
113. Wilcox, C. *et al.* 'Using expert elicitation to estimate the impacts of plastic pollution on marine wildlife', *Marine Policy* 65: 107–114 (2015)
114. Ritchie, H. 'The world now produces more seafood from fish farms than wild catch', *Our World in Data,* September 2019, https://ourworldindata.org/rise-of-aquaculture
115. Fry, J. 'Feed conversion efficiency in aquaculture: Do we measure it correctly?' *Environmental Research Letters* 13 (2018)
116. Poore, J., Nemecek, T., 'Reducing food's environmental impacts through producers and consumers'.
117. *Ibid.*
118. Yang, P. *et al.* 'Large contribution of non-aquaculture period fluxes to the annual N2O emissions from aquaculture ponds in Southeast China', *Journal of Hydrology* 582: 124550 (2020)
119. Poore, J., Nemecek, T., 'Reducing food's environmental impacts through producers and consumers'.
120. Thorstad, E. B., Finstad, B. 'Impacts of salmon lice emanating from salmon farms on wild Atlantic salmon and sea trout', NINA report 1449: 1–22 (2018)
121. Searchinger, T. *et al.* 'World Resources Report: Creating a Sustainable Food Future' (World Resources Institute, 2019)

122. *Ibid.*
123. *Ibid.*
124. Carrington, D. 'Avoiding meat and dairy is "single biggest way" to reduce your impact on Earth, *Guardian*, 31 May 2018, https://www.theguardian.com/environment/2018/may/31/avoiding-meat-and-dairy-is-single-biggest-way-to-reduce-your-impact-on-earth

Chapter 5

1. Whitman J. 'Political Processes and Infectious Diseases', in *The Politics of Emerging and Resurgent Infectious Diseases*, (Palgrave Macmillan, 2000)
2. https://www.who.int/news/item/08-12-2010-international-spread-of-disease-threatens-public-health-security
3. Global Preparedness Monitoring Board, 'A world at risk: annual report on global preparedness for health emergencies', (World Health Organization, 2019)
4. Dalton, J. 'Meat-eating creates risk of future pandemics that "would make Covid seem a dress rehearsal", scientists warn', *Independent*, 30 January 2021, https://www.independent.co.uk/climate-change/news/meat-coronavirus-pandemic-science-animals-b1794996.html
5. Schaverien, A. 'The coronavirus pandemic is "not necessarily the big one," senior WHO official says', *The New York Times*, 29 December 2020, https://www.nytimes.com/2020/12/29/world/who-covid-pandemic-big.html
6. Ioannidis, J. P A. 'Infection fatality rate of COVID-19 inferred from seroprevalence data', *Bulletin of the World Health Organization* 99, 1: 19–33F (2021)
7. https://www.cdc.gov/media/pdf/mitigationslides.pdf
8. https://www.cdc.gov/onehealth/basics/zoonotic-diseases.html
9. Food and Agriculture Organization of the United Nations (FAO), World Health Organization (WHO), and World Organisation for Animal Health (OIE), 'Report of the WHO/FAO/OIE joint consultation on emerging zoonotic diseases', (2004)
10. Food and Agriculture Organization of the United Nations (FAO), 'Surge in diseases of animal origin necessitates new approach to health: report' (2013), http://www.fao.org/news/story/en/item/210621/icode/
11. Cyranoski, D. 'Bat cave solves mystery of deadly SARS virus – and suggests new outbreak could occur', *Nature*, 1 December 2017, https://www.nature.com/articles/d41586-017-07766-9
12. Hu, Z. *et al.* 'Identification of Two Critical Amino Acid Residues of the Severe Acute Respiratory Syndrome Coronavirus Spike Protein for Its Variation in Zoonotic Tropism Transition via a Double

Substitution Strategy', *Journal of Biological Chemistry* 280: 29588–95 (2005)

13. https://www.cdc.gov/sars/about/fs-sars.html
14. Farag, E. *et al.* 'Drivers of MERS-CoV Emergence in Qatar', *Viruses* 11, 1: 22 (2018)
15. *Ibid.*
16. https://www.who.int/news-room/fact-sheets/detail/middle-east-res piratory-syndrome-coronavirus-(mers-cov)
17. https://www.who.int/health-topics/middle-east-respiratory-syndrome-coronavirus-mers
18. 'Saudi Arabia: Farmers flout Mers warning by kissing camels', BBC, 13 May 2014, https://www.bbc.co.uk/news/blogs-news-from-elsewhere-27393045
19. Xiao, X. *et al.* 'Animal sales from Wuhan wet markets immediately prior to the COVID-19 pandemic', *Scientific Reports* 11 (2021)
20. AP newswire, 'Racism targets Asian food, business during COVID-19 pandemic', *Independent,* 20 December 2020, https://www.independent.co.uk/news/racism-targets-asian-food-business-during-covid19-pandemic-asian-americans-china-virus-food-us-b1776793.html
21. UNODC, 'Wildlife Crime: Pangolin scales, 2020', United Nations Office on Drugs and Crime.
22. Reuters, 'China scientists says SARS-civet cat link prove', 20 January 2007, https://www.reuters.com/article/us-china-sars-idUSPEK23793120061123
23. Cyranoski, D. 'Bat cave solves mystery of deadly SARS virus – and suggests new outbreak could occur', *Nature,* 1 December 2017, https://www.nature.com/articles/d41586-017-07766-9
24. Nuzzo, J. B. *et al. Preparedness for a High Impact Respiratory Pathogen Pandemic* (The Johns Hopkins Center for Health Security, 2019)
25. https://blogs.cdc.gov/publichealthmatters/2018/05/1918-flu
26. *Ibid.*
27. van der Kolk, J. H. 'Role for migratory domestic poultry and/or wild birds in the global spread of avian influenza?' *Veterinary Quarterly* 39, 1: 161–7 (2019)
28. Wolfe, N.D, Dunavan, C.P., Diamond, J. 'Irigins of major human infectious diseases', in Institute of Medicine (US), *Improving Food Safety Through a One Health Approach: Workshop Summary* (National Academies Press, 2012)
29. Corman, V. *et al.* 'Link of a ubiquitous human coronavirus to dromedary camels', Proceedings of the National Academy of Sciences 113 (2016)
30. Martin D. L., Goodman, A. H. 'Health conditions before Columbus: paleopathology of native North Americans', *Western Journal of Medicine* 176, 1: 65–8 (2002)

31. Park, S., Hongu, N., Daily III, J. 'Native American Foods: History, Culture, and Influence on Modern Diets', *Journal of Ethnic Foods* 3 (2016)

32. Marr J. S., Cathey J. T. 'New hypothesis for cause of epidemic among native Americans, New England, 1616–19. *Emerging Infectious Diseases* 16, 2: 281–6 (2010)

33. Subbarao, K., Katz, J. 'Avian influenza viruses infecting humans', *Cellular and Molecular Life Sciences* 57: 1770–84 (2000)

34. *Ibid.*

35. Barry J. M. 'The site of origin of the 1918 influenza pandemic and its public health implications'. *Journal of Translational Medicine* 2, 1: 3 (2004)

36. Saul, J. 'Geographical and Biological Origin of the Influenza Pandemic of 1918', *Life: The Excitement of Biology* 6: 5–12 (2018)

37. Nelson, M. I., Worobey, M., 'Origins of the 1918 Pandemic: Revisiting the Swine "Mixing Vessel" Hypothesis', *American Journal of Epidemiology* 187, 12: 2498–2502 (2018)

38. Walters, M. J. 'Birds, Pigs and People: The Rise of Pandemic Flus', *Seven Modern Plagues*: 151–173 (2014)

39. https://www.cdc.gov/flu/pandemic-resources/2009-h1n1-pandemic.html

40. de Jong, M.D. *et al.* 'Fatal avian influenza A (H5N1) in a child presenting with diarrhea followed by coma', *New England Journal of Medicine* 17, 352(7): 686–91 (2005)

41. Marschall, J., Hartmann, K. 'Avian influenza A H5N1 infections in cats', *Journal of Feline Medicine and Surgery* 10, 4: 359–65 (2008)

42. https://www.who.int/influenza/human_animal_interface/2020_10_07_tableH5N1.pdf

43. Nuzzo, J. B. *et al. Preparedness for a High Impact Respiratory Pathogen Pandemic* (The Johns Hopkins Center for Health Security, 2019)

44. Li, F. C. *et al.* 'Finding the real case-fatality rate of H5N1 avian influenza', *Journal of Epidemiol Community Health* 62, 6: 555–9 (2008)

45. Abdelwhab, E. M., Hafez, H. M. 'Insight into alternative approaches for control of avian influenza in poultry, with emphasis on highly pathogenic H5N1', *Viruses* 4, 11: 3179–3208 (2012)

46. Spiress, A. 'Bird flu drug rendered useless', *Washington Post,* 18 June 2005, https://www.washingtonpost.com/archive/politics/2005/06/18/bird-flu-drug-rendered-useless/80ffc0a9-c9f7-4cc4-80e7-55bb81fec88a/

47. https://www.cdc.gov/flu/avianflu/h7n9-virus.htm

48. https://www.gov.uk/government/publications/avian-influenza-a-h7n9-public-health-england-risk-assessment/risk-assessment-of-avian-influenza-ah7n9-sixth-update

49. Reuters, 'Philippines ban poultry products from Australia over bird flu outbreak', 19 August 2020, https://www.reuters.com/article/us-philippines-birdflu-australia-idUSKCN25F0FH

50. DEFRA, 'Highly pathogenic avian influenza (HPAI) in the UK, and Europe', 31 March 2021, https://assets.publishing.service.gov.uk/government/uploads/system/uploads/attachment_data/file/975740/Highly_pathogenic_avian_influenza__HPAI__in_the_UK__and_Europe__31_March_2021_.pdf

51. Reuters, 'China confirms first human case of H10N3 bird flu strain', *Guardian*, 1 June 2021, https://www.theguardian.com/world/2021/jun/01/china-confirms-first-human-case-h10n3-bird-flu-strain-man-jiangsu

52. Boyle, L. 'New York City urged to shut down 80 live animal markets amid fresh pandemic fears', *Independent*, 7 May 2020, https://www.independent.co.uk/climate-change/news/new-york-live-animal-wet-market-coronavirus-wildlife-pandemic-disease-a9500796.html

53. Dhingra, M. S. *et al*. 'Geographical and Historical Patterns in the Emergences of Novel Highly Pathogenic Avian Influenza (HPAI) H5 and H7 Viruses in Poultry', *Frontiers in Veterinary Science 5*, 84 (2018)

54. Olsen, S. J. *et al*. 'Estimating Risk to Responders Exposed to Avian Influenza A H5 and H7 Viruses in Poultry, United States, 2014–2017', *Emerging Infectious Diseases 25*, 5: 1011–14 (2019)

55. World Health Organization, *Avian Influenza: Assessing the Pandemic Threat* (World Health Organization, 2005) https://apps.who.int/iris/bitstream/handle/10665/68985/WHO_CDS_2005.29.pdf?sequence=1&isAllowed=y

56. Taylor D. 'Seeing the forests for the more than the trees', *Environmental Health Perspectives 105*, 11: 1186–91 (1997)

57. Zimmer, K. 'Deforestation is leading to more infectious diseases in humans', *National Geographic*, 22 November 2019, https://www.nationalgeographic.com/science/article/deforestation-leading-to-more-infectious-diseases-in-humans

58. Steinfeld, H. 'Livestock's Long Shadow: Environmental Issues and Options', Rome: Food and Agriculture Organization of the United Nations (2006)

59. Murray K. A. *et al*. 'Emerging Viral Zoonoses from Wildlife Associated with Animal-Based Food Systems: Risks and Opportunities', in Jay-Russell M., Doyle M. (eds) *Food Safety Risks from Wildlife* (Springer, 2016)

60. https://globalforestcoalition.org/wp-content/uploads/2016/12/bolivia-case-study.pdf

61. De Sy, V. *et al*. 'Land use patterns and related carbon losses following deforestation in South America', *Environmental Research Letters 10*: 124004 (2015)

62. Veiga, C. 'Deforestation sparks yellow fever outbreak in Brazil', *Dialogo Chino*, 10 February 2017, https://dialogochino.net/en/agriculture/8488-deforestation-sparks-yellow-fever-outbreak-in-brazil
63. Steinfeld, H. 'Livestock's Long Shadow: Environmental Issues and Options'.
64. Constable, H. 'The other virus that worries Asia', BBC, 6 January 2021, https://www.bbc.com/future/article/20210106-nipah-virus-how-bats-could-cause-the-next-pandemic
65. https://www.who.int/news-room/fact-sheets/detail/nipah-virus
66. Ritchie, H. 'Cutting down forests: what are the drivers of deforestation', *Our World in Data*, 23 February 2021, https://ourworldindata.org/what-are-drivers-deforestation
67. https://www.who.int/news-room/fact-sheets/detail/ebola-virus-disease
68. https://www.cdc.gov/vhf/ebola/history/2014-2016-outbreak/index.html
69. Onyekuru, N.A., *et al.* 'Effects of Ebola Virus Disease Outbreak on Bush Meat Enterprise and Environmental Health Risk Behavior Among Households in South-East Nigeria', *Journal of Primary Prevention* 41: 603–18 (2020)
70. https://www.avert.org/professionals/history-hiv-aids/origin
71. https://www.unaids.org/en/resources/fact-sheet
72. Omoleke, S.A., Mohammed, I., Saidu, Y. 'Ebola Viral Disease in West Africa: A Threat to Global Health, Economy and Political Stability', *Journal of Public Health in Africa* 7, 1 :534 (2016)
73. https://www.un.org/en/chronicle/article/illegal-commercial-bushmeat-trade-central-and-west-africa
74. Chaber, A. *et al.* 'The scale of illegal meat importation from Africa to Europe via Paris', *Conservation Letters* 3: 317–21 (2010)
75. Lynn, G. 'Cane rat meat "sold to public" in Ridley Road market', BBC, 17 September 2012, https://www.bbc.co.uk/news/uk-england-london-19622903
76. Dawson S. 'Bushmeat', *Food Ethics Education* 13: 209–20 (2017)
77. Gombeer, S. *et al.* 'Exploring the bushmeat market in Brussels, Belgium: a clandestine luxury business', *Biodiversity and Conservation* (2021)
78. Flynn, G., Scutti, S. 'Smuggled bushmeat is ebola's back door to America', *Newsweek*, 29 August 2014, https://www.newsweek.com/2014/08/29/smuggled-bushmeat-ebolas-back-door-america-265668.html
79. de Wit, E., Munster, V. J. 'Animal models of disease shed light on Nipah virus pathogenesis and transmission', *Journal of Pathology* 235, 2: 196–205 (2015)
80. Brauburger, K., *et al.* 'Forty-five years of Marburg virus research', *Viruses* 4, 10: 1878–1927 (2012)

81. https://www.worldanimalprotection.org.uk/news/exotic-pets-are-you-willing-pay-price

82. https://www.cdc.gov/poxvirus/monkeypox/outbreak.html

83. https://www.cidrap.umn.edu/news-perspective/2005/11/england-query-quarantined-bird-deaths-implicates-taiwan

84. Green, E. 'Britain details the start of its "Mad Cow" outbreak', *The New York Times,* 26 January 1999, https://www.nytimes.com/1999/01/26/science/britain-details-the-start-of-its-mad-cow-outbreak.html

85. Pickrell, J. 'Timeline: BSE and vCJD', *New Scientist,* 4 September 2006, https://www.newscientist.com/article/dn9926-timeline-bse-and-vcjd

86. https://www.cdc.gov/prions/bse/about.html

87. https://www.theguardian.com/uk/2000/oct/29/bse.focus1

88. ' "Mad cow disease": what is BSE?', BBC, 18 October 2018, https://www.bbc.co.uk/news/uk-45906585

89. http://news.bbc.co.uk/onthisday/hi/dates/stories/may/16/newsid_2913000/2913807.stm

90. 'Government has ruled out BSE link with man's death', *The Herald,* 15 August 1995, https://www.heraldscotland.com/news/1209 1003.government-has-ruled-out-bse-link-with-mans-death

91. 'Madness', *Observer,* 29 October 2000, https://www.theguardian.com/uk/2000/oct/29/bse.focus1

92. *Ibid.*

93. Maheshwari, A., *et al.* 'Recent US Case of Variant Creutzfeldt-Jakob Disease-Global Implications', *Emerging Infectious Diseases* 21, 5: 750–9 (2015)

94. Head, M. W., Ironside, J.W. 'Mad cows and monkey business: the end of vCJD?', *Lancet* 365, 9461: 730–1 (2005)

95. https://www.bmj.com/press-releases/2013/10/14/researchers-estimate-one-2000-people-uk-carry-variant-cjd-proteins

96. Mackenzie, D. 'Many more people could still die from mad cow disease in the UK', *New Scientist,* 18 January 2017, https://www.newscientist.com/article/2118418-many-more-people-could-still-die-from-mad-cow-disease-in-the-uk

97. https://publications.parliament.uk/pa/cm201415/cmselect/cmsctech/327/32707.htm

98. https://publications.parliament.uk/pa/cm201415/cmselect/cmsctech/327/32707.htm

99. https://www.gov.uk/guidance/supplying-and-using-animal-by-products-as-farm-animal-feed

100. https://www.govinfo.gov/content/pkg/FR-2008-04-25/html/08-1180.htm

101. Greger, M. 'Mad cow California: stop weaning calves on cattle blood', *Huffpost,* 25 April 2012, https://www.huffpost.com/entry/california-mad-cow-disease_b_1450984

102. Holland. D, *et al*. 'Estimating deaths from foodborne disease in the UK for 11 key pathogens', *BMJ Open Gastroenterology* 7, 1 (2020)

103. Lawrence, F. 'Three-quarters of supermarket chickens contaminated with campylobacter', *Guardian*, 28 May 2015, https://www.theguardian.com/lifeandstyle/2015/may/28/supermarket-chickens-contaminated-campylobacter

104. *Ibid*.

105. Whitworth, J. J. 'FSA reverses Campylobacter names and shame plan', *Food Navigator*, 23 July 2014, https://www.foodnavigator.com/Article/2014/07/24/FSA-backs-down-on-Campylobacter-testing-results

106. Goodley, S. 'UK's top supplier of supermarket chicken fiddles food safety dates', *Guardian*, 28 September 2017, https://www.theguardian.com/business/2017/sep/28/uks-top-supplier-of-supermarket-chicken-fiddles-food-safety-dates

107. https://www.cdc.gov/foodborneburden/2011-foodborne-estimates.html

108. Levitt, T., Kendall, L. ' "Unacceptable" bacteria levels found on US meat may fuel fears over UK trade deal', *Guardian*, 10 October 2020, https://www.theguardian.com/environment/2020/oct/10/unacceptable-bacteria-levels-found-on-us-meat-may-fuel-fears-over-uk-trade-deal

109. Barry, D. 'Turkey, glue and you', *Washington Post*, 5 November 1995, https://www.washingtonpost.com/archive/lifestyle/magazine/1995/11/05/turkey-glue-and-you/b22d658f-72fe-4a5c-944f-ec6111d18042/

110. Prior, R. 'It's legal for your meat to have trace amounts of fecal matter. A group of doctors want to change that', *CNN*, 17 April 2019, https://edition.cnn.com/2019/04/17/health/usda-fecal-matter-in-meat-trnd/index.html

111. Carr, T. 'Unclean greens: how America's E-coli outbreaks in salads are linked to cows', *Guardian*, 1 September 2020, https://www.theguardian.com/environment/2020/sep/01/unclean-greens-how-americas-e-coli-outbreaks-in-salads-are-linked-to-cows

112. https://www.who.int/news-room/fact-sheets/detail/antibiotic-resistance

113. Kirchhelle, C. 'Pharming animals: a global history of antibiotics in food production (1935–2017)', *Palgrave Commununications* 4, 96 (2018)

114. *Ibid*.

115. *Ibid*.

116. Stolberg, S. G. 'Superbugs', *The New York Times* magazine, 2 August 1998, https://www.nytimes.com/1998/08/02/magazine/superbugs.html

117. Burros, M. 'Poultry industry quietly cuts back on antibiotic use', *The New York Times*, 10 February 2002, https://www.nytimes.

com/2002/02/10/us/poultry-industry-quietly-cuts-back-on-antibiotic-use.html

118. Compassion in World Farming, 'Why the use of fluoroquinolone antibiotics in poultry should be banned', April 2016, https://www.ciwf.org.uk/media/7427394/why-the-use-of-fluoroquinolone-antibiotics-in-poultry-must-be-banned.pdf

119. Wasley, A., Parsons, V. 'Poultry farmers "using more antibiotics linked to resistant food poisoning bugs"', *Independent,* 7 February 2016,https://www.independent.co.uk/life-style/health-and-families/health-news/poultry-farmers-using-more-antibiotics-linked-resistant-food-poisoning-bugs-a6859436.html

120. Wasley, A., Levitt, T., Savage, S. 'UK pig farms doubled their use of class of antibiotics vital for humans', *Guardian,* 17 June 2021, https://www.theguardian.com/environment/2021/jun/17/uk-pig-farms-doubled-their-use-of-antibiotics-vital-for-humans

121. Wasley, A., Parsons, V. 'Poultry farmers "using more antibiotics linked to resistant food poisoning bugs"'

122. Alliance to Save Our Antibiotics, 'Evidence of serious misuse of antibiotics in farmed animals in US, Australia, New Zealand and Canada exposes public health threat of trade deals', 2020, https://www.saveourantibiotics.org/news/press-release/evidence-of-serious-misuse-of-antibiotics-in-farmed-animals-in-us-australia-new-zealand-and-canada-exposes-public-health-threat-of-trade-deals

123. Ritchie, H. 'How do we reduce antibiotic resistance from livestock?', *Our World in Data,* 16 November 2017, https://ourworldindata.org/antibiotic-resistance-from-livestock

124. Harvey, F. 'India's farmed chickens dosed with world's strongest antibiotics, study finds', *Guardian,* 1 February 2018, https://www.theguardian.com/environment/2018/feb/01/indias-farmed-chickens-dosed-with-worlds-strongest-antibiotics-study-finds

125. https://www.who.int/news/item/29-04-2019-new-report-calls-for-urgent-action-to-avert-antimicrobial-resistance-crisis

126. Review on Antimicrobial Resistance, 'Antimicrobial Resistance: Tackling a Crisis for the Health and Wealth of Nations', 2014

127. https://www.who.int/health-topics/cancer

128. United Nations Environment Programme and International Livestock Research Institute, 'Preventing the Next Pandemic: Zoonotic diseases and how to break the chain of transmission', 6 July 2020.

Chapter 6

1. Craig, W. J., Mangels, A. R., American Dietetic Association, 'Position of the American Dietetic Association: vegetarian diets', *Journal of the American Dietetic Association* 109, 7: 1266–82 (2009)

ENDNOTES

2. https://www.bda.uk.com/resource/vegetarian-vegan-plant-based-diet.html
3. https://www.nhs.uk/live-well/eat-well/the-vegan-diet
4. https://www.health.harvard.edu/staying-healthy/becoming-a-vegetarian
5. https://www.mayoclinic.org/healthy-lifestyle/nutrition-and-healthy-eating/in-depth/art-20046446
6. American Dietetic Association, Dietitians of Canada, 'Position of the American Dietetic Association and Dietitians of Canada: Vegetarian diets', *Journal of the American Dietetic Association* 103, 6: 748–65, (2003)
7. Quagliani, D., Felt-Gunderson, P. 'Closing America's Fiber Intake Gap: Communication Strategies from a Food and Fiber Summit', *American Journal of Lifestyle Medicine* 11, 1: 80–5 (2016)
8. Gallagher, J. 'The lifesaving food 90% aren't eating enough of', BBC, 11 January 2019, https://www.bbc.co.uk/news/health-46827426
9. DiNicolantonio, J. J., O'Keefe, J. H., Wilson, W. 'Subclinical magnesium deficiency: a principal driver of cardiovascular disease and a public health crisis', *Open Heart* 5, 1 (2018) [published correction appears in *Open Heart* 5, 5]
10. Southey, F., '"To B12 or Not to B12": The Vegan Society slams "misleading" advert promoting meat and dairy', *Food Navigator,* 11 February 2021, https://www.foodnavigator.com/Article/2021/02/11/The-Vegan-Society-complains-to-ASA-for-misleading-ADHB-advert
11. Willett, W. *et al.* 'Food in the Anthropocene: the EAT-Lancet Commission on healthy diets from sustainable food systems', *Lancet* 393, 10170: 447–92 (2019) [correction appears in *Lancet* 393, 10171: 530; and 393, 10191: 2590; and 395, 10221: 338; and 396, 10256: e56]
12. Carrington, D. 'New plant-focused diet would "transform" planet's future, say scientists', *Guardian,* 16 January 2019, https://www.theguardian.com/environment/2019/jan/16/new-plant-focused-diet-would-transform-planets-future-say-scientists
13. *Ibid.*
14. https://www.bluezones.com/#section-2
15. Crimarco, A. *et al.* 'A randomized crossover trial on the effect of plant-based compared with animal-based meat on trimethylamine-N-oxide and cardiovascular disease risk factors in generally healthy adults: Study With Appetizing Plantfood—Meat Eating Alternative Trial (SWAP-MEAT)', *American Journal of Clinical Nutrition* 112, 5: 1188–99 (2020)
16. Toribio-Mateas MA, Bester A, Klimenko N. 'Impact of Plant-Based Meat Alternatives on the Gut Microbiota of Consumers: A Real-World Study', *Foods.* 10, 9:2040 (2021)

17. Public Health England, 'Government Dietary Recommendations Government recommendations for energy and nutrients for males and females aged 1–18 years and 19+ years', 2016, https://assets. publishing.service.gov.uk/government/uploads/system/uploads/attachment_data/file/618167/government_dietary_recommendations.pdf

18. Huang, J., *et al.* 'Association Between Plant and Animal Protein Intake and Overall and Cause-Specific Mortality', *JAMA Internal Medicine* 180, 9: 1173–84 (2020)

19. Naghshi, S. 'Dietary intake of total, animal, and plant proteins and risk of all cause, cardiovascular, and cancer mortality: Systematic review and dose-response meta-analysis of prospective cohort studies', *British Medical Journal* 370, m2412 (2020)

20. Mangano, K. M. *et al.* 'Dietary protein is associated with musculoskeletal health independently of dietary pattern: the Framingham Third Generation Study', *American Journal of Clinical Nutrition* 105, 3: 714–22 (2017)

21. Longo, U. G. *et al.* 'The Best Athletes in Ancient Rome were Vegetarian!', *Journal of Sports Science Medicine* 7, 4: 565 (2008)

22. Bastide, N. M., Pierre, F. H., Corpet, D. E. 'Heme iron from meat and risk of colorectal cancer: a meta-analysis and a review of the mechanisms involved', *Cancer Prevention Research* 4, 2: 177–84 (2011)

23. Cross, A. J., Pollock, J. R., Bingham, S. A., 'Haem, not protein or inorganic iron, is responsible for endogenous intestinal N-nitrosation arising from red meat', *Cancer Research* 63, 10: 2358–60 (2003)

24. Zhu, Y. *et al.* 'Dietary N-nitroso compounds and risk of colorectal cancer: a case-control study in Newfoundland and Labrador and Ontario, Canada', *British Journal of Nutrition* 111, 6: 1109–17 (2014)

25. Fang, X. *et al.* 'Dietary intake of heme iron and risk of cardiovascular disease: a dose-response meta-analysis of prospective cohort studies', Nutrition Metabolism Cardiovascular Disease 25, 1: 24–35 (2015)

26. https://www.nhs.uk/conditions/vitamins-and-minerals/iron

27. Shin, J., *et al.* 'Effect of Plant- and Animal-Based Foods on Prostate Cancer Risk', *Journal of the American Osteopathic Association* (2019)

28. Ganmaa, D. *et al.* 'Incidence and mortality of testicular and prostatic cancers in relation to world dietary practices', *International Journal of Cancer* 98, 2: 262–7 (2002)

29. Ding, M. *et al.* 'Associations of dairy intake with risk of mortality in women and men: Three prospective cohort studies', *British Medical Journal* 367, l6204 (2019)

30. Burckhardt, P. 'Calcium revisited, part III: effect of dietary calcium on BMD and fracture risk', *BoneKEy Reports* 4: 708 (2015)
31. Tesco, 'Encouraging sustainable feeding practices in the aquaculture industry', August 2019, https://www.tescoplc.com/updates/2019/encouraging-sustainable-feeding-practices-in-the-aquaculture-industry/
32. https://ods.od.nih.gov/factsheets/VitaminB12-HealthProfessional
33. https://www.sentienceinstitute.org/us-factory-farming-estimates
34. https://www.crnusa.org/newsroom/dietary-supplement-usage-increases-says-new-survey
35. https://www.food.gov.uk/sites/default/files/media/document/food-supplements-consumer-research.pdf
36. https://www.cdc.gov/chronicdisease/resources/infographic/chronic-diseases.htm
37. 'Number of Britons living chronic illnesses set to rise', *Guardian*, 24 January 2018, https://www.theguardian.com/society/2018/jan/24/number-of-britons-living-with-chronic-illnesses-set-to-rise
38. https://www.who.int/news-room/fact-sheets/detail/the-top-10-causes-of-death
39. https://www.cdc.gov/heartdisease/facts.htm
40. Dai, H. *et al*. 'Global, regional, and national burden of ischemic heart disease and its attributable risk factors, 1990z–2017: results from the global Burden of Disease Study 2017', *European Heart Journal Quality Care Clinical Outcomes* (2020)
41. Yokoyama, Y., Levin, S. M., Barnard, N. D. 'Association between plant-based diets and plasma lipids: a systematic review and meta-analysis', *Nutritional Review* 75, 9: 683–98 (2017)
42. Esselstyn, C. B. *et al*. 'A way to reverse CAD?', *Journal of Family Practice* 63, 7: 356–64b (2014)
43. Virani, S. S. *et al*. 'Heart Disease and Stroke Statistics—2020 Update: A Report from the American Heart Association', the American Heart Association Council on Epidemiology and Prevention Statistics Committee and Stroke Statistics Subcommittee
44. Baden, M. Y. *et al*. 'Quality of Plant-Based Diet and Risk of Total, Ischemic, and Hemorrhagic Stroke', *Neurology* 96, 15 (2021)
45. Tong, T. Y. N. *et al*. 'Risks of ischaemic heart disease and stroke in meat eaters, fish eaters, and vegetarians over 18 years of follow-up: results from the prospective EPIC-Oxford study', *British Medical Journal* 366: l4897 (2019)
46. https://www.bmj.com/content/bmj/suppl/2019/09/04/bmj.l4897.DC1/tont046481.ww.pdf
47. Appleby, P. N. *et al*. 'Mortality in vegetarians and comparable non-vegetarians in the United Kingdom', *American Journal of Clinical Nutrition* 103, 1: 218–30 (2016)

48. He, F. J., Nowson, C. A., MacGregor, G. A. 'Fruit and vegetable consumption and stroke: meta-analysis of cohort studies', *Lancet* 367, 9507: 320–6 (2006)

49. Carlsen, M. H., *et al.* 'The total antioxidant content of more than 3100 foods, beverages, spices, herbs and supplements used worldwide', *Nutrition Journal* 9, 3 (2010)

50. Rautiainen, S., *et al.* 'Total antioxidant capacity of diet and risk of stroke: a population-based prospective cohort of women', *Stroke* 43, 2: 335–40 (2012)

51. Lee-Kwan, S. H. *et al.* 'Disparities in State-Specific Adult Fruit and Vegetable Consumption—United States, 2015', *Morbidity and Mortality Weekly Report* 66: 1241–7 (2017), https://www.cdc.gov/mmwr/volumes/66/wr/mm6645a1.htm?s_cid=mm6645a1_w

52. https://www.alz.org/aaic/releases_2019/sunLIFESTYLE-jul14.asp

53. LaMotte, S. 'Mediterranean style diet may prevent dementia', CNN, 17 July 2018, https://edition.cnn.com/2017/07/17/health/mediterranean-style-diet-prevents-dementia/index.html

54. Sáiz-Vazquez, O. *et al.* 'Cholesterol and Alzheimer's Disease Risk: A Meta-Meta-Analysis', *Brain Science* 10, 6: 386 (2020)

55. Liang, Y. *et al.* 'Cardiovascular health metrics from mid- to late-life and risk of dementia: A population-based cohort study in Finland', *PLoS Medicine* 17, 12 (2020)

56. Sabia, S. *et al.* 'Association of ideal cardiovascular health at age 50 with incidence of dementia: 25 Year follow-up of Whitehall II cohort study', *British Medical Journal* 366, l4414 (2019)

57. Solomon, A. *et al.* 'Midlife Serum Cholesterol and Increased Risk of Alzheimer's and Vascular Dementia Three Decades Later', *Dementia and Geriatric Cognitive Disorders* 28: 75–80 (2009)

58. Huang, W. J., Zhang, X., Chen, W. W. 'Role of oxidative stress in Alzheimer's disease', *Biomedical Reports* 4, 5: 519–22 (2016)

59. Shishtar, E. *et al.* 'Long-term dietary flavonoid intake and risk of Alzheimer disease and related dementias in the Framingham Offspring Cohort', *American Journal of Clinical* Nutrition 112, 2: 343–53 (2020)

60. Barnard, N. D. *et al.* 'Dietary and lifestyle guidelines for the prevention of Alzheimer's disease', *Neurobiological Aging* 35, suppl 2: S74–8 (2014)

61. https://www.diabetes.org.uk/professionals/position-statements-reports/statistics

62. McMacken, M, Shah, S. 'A plant-based diet for the prevention and treatment of type 2 diabetes', *Journal of Geriatric Cardiology* 14, 5: 342–54 (2017)

63. Fraser, G. E. 'Vegetarian diets: what do we know of their effects on common chronic diseases?' *American Journal of Clinical Nutrition*

89, 5: 1607S-12S (2009) [correction appears in *American Journal of Clinical Nutrition* 90, 1: 248]

64. Emil, M. *et al.* 'Plant-based diet according to the NFI protocol in patients with type 2 diabetes mellitus: pilot study', 2020.

65. Mitchell, K. 'Insurance company to prescribe NFI protocol to "thousands" of T2 diabetes patients', *Plant Based News,* 2 September 2020, https://plantbasednews.org/lifestyle/insurance-company-prescribe-nfi-diet-t2-diabetes-patients

66. Bouvard, V., International Agency for Research on Cancer Monograph Working Group, *et al.* 'Carcinogenicity of consumption of red and processed meat', *Lancet Oncology* 16, 16: 1599–600 (2015)

67. T.H. Chan School of Public Health, Harvard, 'WHO report says eating processed meat is carcinogenic: understanding the findings', 3 November 2015, https://www.hsph.harvard.edu/nutritionsource/2015/11/03/report-says-eating-processed-meat-is-carcinogenic-understanding-the-findings

68. Boseley, S. 'Processed meats rank alongside smoking as cancer causes – WHO', *Guardian,* 26 October 2015, https://www.theguardian.com/society/2015/oct/26/bacon-ham-sausages-processed-meats-cancer-risk-smoking-says-who

69. Arnold, M. *et al.* 'Global patterns and trends in colorectal cancer incidence and mortality' *Gut* 66: 683–91 (2017)

70. *Ibid.*

71. Tabung, F. K. *et al.* 'Association of Dietary Inflammatory Potential with Colorectal Cancer Risk in Men and Women', *JAMA Oncology* 4, 3: 366–73 (2018)

72. Allen, N. E. *et al.* 'The Associations of Diet with Serum Insulin-like Growth Factor I and Its Main Binding Proteins in 292 Women Meat-Eaters, Vegetarians, and Vegans', *Cancer Epidemiology, Biomarkers and Prevention* 11, 11: 1441–8 (2002)

73. Travis, R. C. *et al.* on behalf of the Endogenous Hormones, Nutritional Biomarkers and Prostate Cancer Collaborative Group, 'A Meta-analysis of Individual Participant Data Reveals an Association between Circulating Levels of IGF-I and Prostate Cancer Risk', *Cancer Research* 76, 8: 2288–300 (2016)

74. Murphy, N. *et al.* 'Insulin-like growth factor-1, insulin-like growth factor-binding protein-3, and breast cancer risk: observational and Mendelian randomization analyses with ~430 000 women', *Annals of Oncology* 31, 5: 641–9 (2020)

75. Okekunle, A. *et al.* 'Higher dietary soy intake appears inversely related to breast cancer risk independent of estrogen receptor breast cancer phenotypes', *Heliyon* 6, 7 (2020)

76. Applegate C. C. *et al.* 'Soy Consumption and the Risk of Prostate Cancer: An Updated Systematic Review and Meta-Analysis', *Nutrients* 10, 1: 40 (2018)

77. Reed, K. E. *et al.* 'Neither soy nor isoflavone intake affects male reproductive hormones: An expanded and updated meta-analysis of clinical studies', *Reproductive Toxicology* 100:60–67 (2021)

78. Messina, M. 'Soybean isoflavone exposure does not have feminizing effects on men: a critical examination of the clinical evidence', *Fertility and Sterility* 93, 7: 2095-104 (2010)

79. Willett, W. *et al.* 'Food in the Anthropocene: the EAT-Lancet Commission on healthy diets from sustainable food systems'.

80. Carrington, D. 'New plant-focused diet would "transform" planet's future, say scientists', *Guardian*, 16 January 2019, https://www.theguardian.com/environment/2019/jan/16/new-plant-focused-diet-would-transform-planets-future-say-scientists

81. Springmann, M. *et al.* 'Analysis and valuation of the health and climate change cobenefits of dietary change', *Proceedings of the National Academy of Sciences* 113, 15: 4146–51 (2016)

82. Tuso, MD, P. J. *et al.* 'Nutritional Update for Physicians: Plant-Based Diets'. *Permanente Journal* 17, 2: 61–6 (2013)

Chapter 7

1. Born, P. 'Regarding Animals: A Perspective on the Importance of Animals in Early Childhood Environmental Education', *International Journal of Early Childhood Environmental Education* 5, 2: 46 (2018)

2. Bennett, J. 'Police shoot dead Daisy the cow after its escape from an abattoir in Carlisle to "protect the public" despite social media users rallying behind the bovine's bid for freedom', *Daily Mail*, 24 August 2019, https://www.dailymail.co.uk/news/article-7379733/Police-shoot-dead-Daisy-cow-escape-abattoir-Carlisle.html

3. https://www.legis.iowa.gov/legislation/BillBook?ga=88&ba=SF2413

4. https://www.animallaw.info/statute/ia-cruelty-injury-animals-other-livestock#s2

5. Dalton, J. 'Cows sexually abused, hit and punched at company owned by NFU deputy president, footage shows', *Independent*, 29 November 2019, https://www.independent.co.uk/climate-change/news/cow-sexual-abuse-violence-dairy-farm-punch-kick-hit-essex-nfu-a9215306.html

6. *Ibid.*

7. Sims, A. 'Gardener jailed for killing nine ducklings with lawnmower', *Independent*, 27 July 2015, https://www.independent.co.uk/news/world/americas/gardener-jailed-killing-nine-ducklings-lawnmower-10419465.html

8. 'Rescued piglets served up as sausages to firefighters', BBC, 23 August 2017, https://www.bbc.co.uk/news/uk-england-wiltshire-41012135

9. Sneddon, L. U. 'Evolution of nociception and pain: evidence from fish models', *Philosophical Transactions of the Royal Society B: Biological Sciences* 374, 1785: 20190290 (2019)

10. Hazel, S. J., O'Dwyer, L., Ryan, T. ' "Chickens Are a Lot Smarter than I Originally Thought": Changes in Student Attitudes to Chickens Following a Chicken Training Class', *Animals 5*, 3: 821–37 (2015)

11. Willsher, K. ' "We love foie gras": French outrage at UK plan to ban imports of "cruel" delicacy, *Guardian,* 17 April 2021, https://www.theguardian.com/environment/2021/apr/17/we-love-foie-gras-french-outrage-uk-plan-import-ban-delicacy

12. Skippon, W. 'The animal health and welfare consequences of foie gras production', *Canadian Veterinary Journal 54,* 4: 403–4 (2013)

13. *Ibid.*

14. Sharman, J. 'Sheep farmer felt so guilty on way to slaughterhouse he drove lambs to sanctuary and became vegetarian', *Independent,* 30 January 2019, https://www.independent.co.uk/news/uk/home-news/sheep-farmer-vegetarian-lambs-sanctuary-slaughter-meat-industry-dairy-devon-a8754056.html

15. 'The Dark Side of Dairy', BBC, 10 September 2018, https://www.bbc.co.uk/news/av/uk-scotland-45439303

16. Forrest, S. 'The troubled history of horse meat in America', *The Atlantic,* 8 June 2017. https://www.theatlantic.com/technology/archive/2017/06/horse-meat/529665

17. https://fsa-catalogue2.s3.eu-west-2.amazonaws.com/foi-response-horses-slaughtered-food-chain.pdf

18. 'Horsemeat: EU imports and exports data', *Guardian,* 13 February 2013, https://www.theguardian.com/news/datablog/2013/feb/13/horsemeat-uk-eu-imports-exports

19. Hickman, M. 'Eaten in Britain until the 1930s – but horsemeat has fallen out of favour', *Independent,* 16 January 2013, https://www.independent.co.uk/news/uk/home-news/eaten-britain-until-1930s-horsemeat-has-fallen-out-favour-8454511.html

20. https://trove.nla.gov.au/newspaper/article/59530720

21. https://timesmachine.nytimes.com/timesmachine/1907/06/23/106756317.pdf

22. Savage, J. 'Dogs and cats "still eaten in Switzerland", *The Local,* 27 December 2012, https://www.thelocal.ch/20121227/dogs-still-eaten-in-switzerland

23. Townsend, S. 'NSW Farmers' change terminology for livestock industry', *The Land,* 30 July 2019, https://www.theland.com.au/story/6291345/farmers-ditch-slaughter-for-public-image

24. https://socialsci.libretexts.org/Bookshelves/Sociology/Introduction_to_Sociology/Book%3A_Sociology_(Boundless)/06%3A_Social_

Groups_and_Organization/6.05%3A_Group_Dynamics/6.5C%
3A_The_Asch_Experiment-_The_Power_of_Peer_Pressure

Chapter 8

1. Street-Porter, J. 'Militant veganism is out of control – how long until there's a Vegan Party begging for our votes?', *Independent*, 24 May 2019, https://www.independent.co.uk/voices/veganism-politics-vegan-party-beliefs-environment-election-climate-change-a8929 271.html
2. 'Farmers "sent death threats by vegan activists"', BBC, 29 January 2018, https://www.bbc.co.uk/news/av/uk-42860384
3. Haque, A. 'Vegans call me murderer and rapist', BBC, 29 January 2018, https://www.bbc.co.uk/news/uk-42833132
4. Chiorando, M. '"Death Threat" Farmer Admits "I've Not Had People Making Specific Death Threats Towards Me"', *Plant Based News*, 7 February 2018, https://plantbasednews.org/culture/farmer-admits-not-had-specific-death-threats-towards-me
5. Chiorando, M. '#Februdairy Leader "Likes" Tweet About "Shooting Vegans"', *Plant Based News*, 7 October 2020, https://plantbasednews.org/news/februdairy-leader-likes-tweet-about-shooting-vegans
6. Robinson, B. 'Vegan activists want farmers children HURT as veggie politics get VERY DARK', *Daily Express*, 3 February 2018, https://www.express.co.uk/news/uk/914062/vegan-diet-activists-target-farmers-hurt-children-allege-animal-abuse-Joey-Armstrong
7. Snowdon, K. 'A Vegan Died on Mount Everest, Papers Are Keen to Tell Us – Not That She Was an Academic, A Wife, And an Experienced Climber', *Huffpost*, 23 May 2016, https://www.huffingtonpost.co.uk/kathryn-snowdon/a-vegan-died-on-mount-everest_b_10105070.html
8. 'Vegan diet kills baby', *Mirror*, 3 May 2007, https://www.mirror.co.uk/news/uk-news/vegan-diet-kills-baby-471794
9. Glaister, D. 'Parents jailed for death of underfed baby', *Guardian*, 10 May 2007, https://www.theguardian.com/world/2007/may/10/usa.danglaister
10. McCloskey, J. 'Screaming baby starved to death surrounded by curdled milk as mother did nothing', *Metro*, 18 April 2020, https://metro.co.uk/2020/04/18/screaming-baby-starved-death-surrounded-curdled-milk-mother-nothing-12575641
11. Johnston, B. C. *et al.* 'Unprocessed Red Meat and Processed Meat Consumption: Dietary Guideline Recommendations From the Nutritional Recommendations (NutriRECS) Consortium', *Annals of Internal Medicine* 171, 10: 756–64 (2019).

12. Pawlowski, A., Edison, N. 'There's no need to eat less red or processed meat, group says, prompting criticism', NBC News, 30 September 2019, https://www.nbcnews.com/health/heart-health/there-s-no-need-eat-less-red-or-processed-meat-n1060511

13. Swift, D. 'Red Meat OK'd in New Guideline But Critics Call Foul', *Medscape,* 30 September 2019, https://www.medscape.com/viewarticle/919221

14. Parker-Pope, T. and O'Connor, A. 'Scientist Who Discredited Meat Guidelines Didn't Report Past Food Industry Ties', *The New York Times*, 4 October 2019, https://www.nytimes.com/2019/10/04/well/eat/scientist-who-discredited-meat-guidelines-didnt-report-past-food-industry-ties.html

15. https://www.facebook.com/ThisMorning/videos/bacons-back-on-the-menu-study-finds/511629266325367/

16. https://www.bhf.org.uk/what-we-do/news-from-the-bhf/contact-the-press-office/facts-and-figures

17. https://www.bowelcanceruk.org.uk/media

18. You can see the whole exchange at https://www.youtube.com/watch?v=iBL6TxaF5p0&ab_channel=ThisMorning

19. https://www.history.com/news/cigarette-ads-doctors-smoking-endorsement

20. https://meatscience.org/about-amsa

21. https://www.peta.org.uk/features/crappy-eggs-not-happy-eggs

22. Dalton, J. ' "Free-range" hens from Happy Egg suppliers suffer misery in overcrowded sheds, investigators claim', *Independent*, 5 March 2021, https://www.independent.co.uk/news/uk/home-news/free-range-eggs-happy-egg-company-hens-peta-b1812105.html

23. https://cordis.europa.eu/article/id/429495-europe-s-plant-based-food-industry-shows-record-level-growth

24. Giliver, L. 'Vegan Meat Market Grew Twice As Fast As Meat During Pandemic', *Plant Based News,* 6 April 2021, https://plantbasednews.org/news/economics/plant-based-food-sales-exceeded-seven-billion

25. Gleckel, J. A. 'Are Consumers Really Confused by Plant-Based Food Labels? An Empirical Study', University of Louisville, Louis D. Brandeis School of Law, Journal of Animal and Environmental Law (2020)

26. Selyukh, A. 'What Gets to Be a "Burger"? States Restrict Labels on Plant-Based Meat', NPR, 23 July 2019, https://www.npr.org/sections/thesalt/2019/07/23/744083270/what-gets-to-be-a-burger-states-restrict-labels-on-plant-based-meat

27. Moss, M. 'While Warning about Fat, U.S. Pushes Cheese Sales', *The New York Times*, 7 November 2010, https://www.nytimes.com/2010/11/07/us/07fat.html

28. Thielman, S., Rushe, D. 'Government-backed egg lobby tried to crack food startup, emails show', *Guardian,* 2 September 2015, https://www.theguardian.com/us-news/2015/sep/02/usda-american-egg-board-hampton-creek-just-mayo

29. Mohan, G. 'The egg industry launched a secret two-year war against a vegan mayonnaise competitor', *Los Angeles Times,* 7 October 2016, https://www.latimes.com/business/la-fi-egg-board-investigation-20161007-snap-story.html

30. *Ibid.*

31. https://www.agweb.com/news/policy/usda-cracks-down-american-egg-board

32. Lazarus, O., McDermid, S., Jacquet, J. 'The climate responsibilities of industrial meat and dairy producers', *Climatic Change* 165, 30 (2021).

33. https://ahdb.org.uk/news/dairy-industry-unites-to-launch-1m-consumer-campaign

34. https://www.desmog.com/agribusiness-database-agriculture-horticulture-development-board

35. https://www.nutrition.org.uk/aboutbnf/corporate/memberorganisations.html

36. Chiorando, M. 'Dairy Farmers Need "Protection" From Vegan Activists, Says Politician', *Plant Based News,* 26 February 2019, https://plantbasednews.org/culture/dairy-farmers-need-protection-from-vegan-activists

37. Harrison-Dunn, A. 'Ginsters: "manly" ad campaign will fuel male interest', bakeryandsnacks.com, 12 February 2014, https://www.bakeryandsnacks.com/Article/2014/02/12/Ginsters-TV-advert-targets-men-with-manly-campaign

38. Harris, J. 'Carl's Jr. thinks women can't handle its meaty burgers in new ad', *Los Angeles Times*, 9 April 2014, https://www.latimes.com/food/dailydish/la-dd-carls-jr-women-cant-handle-burgers-20140409-story.html

39. 'Burger King advert upsets campaigners', *Guardian,* 7 November 2006, https://www.theguardian.com/media/2006/nov/07/advertising

40. Lockwood, Dr A. 'Could New Advertising Rules On Gender Stereotypes Help Animals?', *Plant Based News,* 18 June 2019, https://plantbasednews.org/opinion/advertising-rules-gender-help-animals

41. Pohlmann, A. 'Men routinely incorporate red meat to preempt the negative emotional states caused by threats to masculinity', Experiment, 6 September 2018, https://experiment.com/projects/meat-can-manhood-stomach-the-punch-of-the-vegetarian-alternative

42. Chiorando, M. ' "Eating Meat Reinforces Toxic Masculinity" According to Academic on Fox News', *Plant Based News,* 20 December 2017, https://plantbasednews.org/culture/eating-meat-reinforces-toxic-masculinity

43. Chan, E., Zlatevska, N. 'Jerkies, Tacos, and Burgers: Subjective Socioeconomic Status and Meat Preference', *Appetite* (2018)
44. Ives, L. 'Deprived areas "have five times more fast food outlets"', BBC, 29 June 2018, https://www.bbc.co.uk/news/health-44642027
45. https://www.rgs.org/about/press-and-media/recent-press-releases/meat-free-men-men-want-to-eat-less-meat-but-avoid
46. Kristiansen, S., Painter, J., Shea, M. 'Animal Agriculture and Climate Change in the US and UK Elite Media: Volume, Responsibilities, Causes and Solutions', *Environmental Communication* 15, 2: 153–72 (2021)
47. *Ibid.*
48. Steinfeld, H. 'Livestock's Long Shadow: Environmental Issues and Options', Food and Agriculture Organization of the United Nations', 2006.
49. https://assets.publishing.service.gov.uk/government/uploads/system/uploads/attachment_data/file/996575/Climate_change_and_net_zero_public_awareness_and_perceptions_summary_report.pdf
50. https://www.desmog.com/2021/07/18/investigation-meat-industry-greenwash-climatewash/
51. Cockburn, H. '"Distressed" farmers condemn Tesco vegetarian advert and suggest teenage girls should eat more meat', *Independent,* 17 October 2019, https://www.independent.co.uk/climate-change/news/nfu-complaint-tesco-vegetarian-range-meat-farmers-teenage-girls-climate-change-a9160181.html
52. Giliver, L. 'BBC Christmas Advert Branded an "Agenda Against Livestock Farming"', *Plant Based News,* 8 December 2019, https://plantbasednews.org/culture/bbc-christmas-advert-branded-agenda-against-livestock-farming

Chapter 9

1. https://www.nationalchickencouncil.org/americans-eat-1-35-billion-chicken-wings-super-bowl
2. https://www.sentienceinstitute.org/us-factory-farming-estimates
3. https://www.nationalchickencouncil.org/americans-eat-1-35-billion-chicken-wings-super-bowl
4. Fuller, A. 'Half of Brits worry about trying to cater to everyone's dietary needs when hosting a barbecue', *Sun*, 13 August 2020, https://www.thesun.co.uk/news/12394253/half-brits-worry-cater-dietary-needs-bbq
5. Gorvett, Z. 'The hidden biases that drive anti-vegan hatred', BBC, 3 February 2020, https://www.bbc.com/future/article/20200203-the-hidden-biases-that-drive-anti-vegan-hatred

6. *Ibid.*
7. Shaw, J. 'What the "meat paradox" reveals about moral decision making', BBC, 6 February 2019, https://www.bbc.com/future/article/20190206-what-the-meat-paradox-reveals-about-moral-decision-making
8. Veilleux, S. 'Coping With Dissonance: Psychological Mechanisms That Enable Ambivalent Attitudes Toward Animals' (2014). University of Maine, Honors College 196 (2014)
9. Mitchell, D. 'My beef with vegans says more about me than them', *Guardian*, 9 December 2018, https://www.theguardian.com/commentisfree/2018/dec/09/my-beef-with-vegans-says-more-about-me-than-them-david-mitchell

Afterword

1. Carrington, D. '$1m a minute: the farming subsidies destroying the world – report', *Guardian*, 16 September 2019, https://www.theguardian.com/environment/2019/sep/16/1m-a-minute-the-farming-subsidies-destroying-the-world
2. https://earth.org/how-costa-rica-reversed-deforestation
3. 'Feeding the Problem: the dangerous intensification of animal farming in Europe', Greenpeace, 12 February 2019, https://www.greenpeace.org/eu-unit/issues/nature-food/1803/feeding-problem-dangerous-intensification-animal-farming
4. Abboud, L. 'UK farmers prepare for overhaul to farm subsidies after Brexit', *Financial Times*, 6 October 2018, https://www.ft.com/content/db2a28e2-c175-11e8-95b1-d36dfef1b89a
5. Dorning, M. 'U.S. farm profit on track for seven-year high after Trump aid', *Bloomberg*, 2 December 2020, https://www.bloomberg.com/news/articles/2020-12-02/u-s-farm-profit-on-track-for-seven-year-high-after-trump-aid?sref=UTbvKgk5
6. Carrington, D. 'Taxing red meat would save many lives, research shows', *Guardian*, 6 November 2018, https://www.theguardian.com/environment/2018/nov/06/taxing-red-meat-would-save-many-lives-research-shows
7. Pieper, M., Michalke, A., Gaugler, T. 'Calculation of external climate costs for food highlights inadequate pricing of animal products', *Nature Communications* 11, 6117 (2020)
8. Bratman, G., *et al.* 'Nature and mental health: An ecosystem service perspective', *Science Advances* 5 (2019)
9. https://businesswales.gov.wales/farmingconnect/sites/farmingconnect/files/technical_article_-_vertical_farming_final.pdf
10. Stein, E. W. 'The Transformative Environmental Effects Large-Scale Indoor Farming May Have on Air, Water, and Soil', *Air, Soil and Water Research* 14, 1 (2021)

11. Carrington, D. 'No-kill, lab-grown meat to go on sale for first time', *Guardian*, 2 December 2020, https://www.theguardian.com/environment/2020/dec/02/no-kill-lab-grown-meat-to-go-on-sale-for-first-time

INDEX

breast cancer 184
breeding buddy 58
Brevig Mission 134–5
Brexit 257
British Dietetic Association 160
British Egg Industry Council
    (BEIC) 54
British Meat Processors
    Association 50
British Medical Journal 150
British Nutrition
    Association 223
broiler chicken 34–5, 74, 78, 139
BSE (bovine spongiform
    encephalopathy) 50, 114–15,
    148–51
Bureau of Investigative Journalism
    43, 56, 91
bushmeat 146–8
bycatch 123, 124, 125

calcium 80, 161, 168–70, 174,
    183, 248
calves
    rearing of 64–5, 70, 71, 72
    separation of young from
        mothers 24, 64–6, 68, 69, 71,
        72, 199
Camp Funston military facility,
    Kansas 138
campylobacter 152, 155
cancer 77, 90, 142, 156, 157, 161,
    167, 168–9, 182–4, 186, 211,
    212, 214
Capper, Jude 209
carbohydrates 30, 31, 63, 181
carbon dioxide emissions 103, 104,
    105, 106, 107, 108, 109–11,
    118, 123–4, 125, 126, 127,
    256
Cargill 50
carnism 244
castration 14, 33, 41, 60, 70, 71, 83
cattle 34, 40, 42, 43, 64–73
    BSE and 50, 114–15, 148–51

calves, rearing of 64–5, 70, 71, 72
calves separation of young from
    mothers 24, 64–6, 68, 69, 71,
    72, 199
calves shot and discarded 70–1
dairy industry and meat
    industry, links between 67,
    69–70
disease and 50, 114–15, 148–51
feedlots 44, 72
foot-and-mouth disease 114–15
grass-fed 109–10
greenhouse gases and 104, 110
group housing 68
impregnation process 64–5
land use and 102, 115, 146, 256
lifespan 66–7
local animal products and 105–7
male calves 68–9
marketing 219, 220
pregnant cow brought to
    slaughter 67–8
selectively bred 34, 66
slaughter of 66–8, 69
solitary confinement hutches 68
veal 68–70, 72, 154, 202
zero-grazing systems 66
censorship, plant-based products
    and 218–20
Centers for Disease Control and
    Prevention (CDC) 143, 153,
    179
Chicken Run 189
chickens 13, 74–81
    animal welfare standards and
        53, 54, 56–7
    barns 75–7, 79
    battery cages 41
    broiler chicken 34–5, 74, 78,
        139
    castration process 41
    cerebral cortex, removal of 45
    'Chicken of Tomorrow' contest
        34–5
    contractors 42–3

INDEX

INDEX

INDEX

INDEX

Food and Agriculture
Organization (FAO) 130
'Livestock's Long Shadow'
report (2006) 229–30
United States Department of
Agriculture (USDA) 34–5, 38,
39, 45, 66, 73, 221, 222
University of Hawaii 225
University of Oxford 101, 102,
108, 185–6
urinary-tract infections (UTIs) 156

vaccination 40–1, 75
veal 68–70, 72, 154, 202
vegan diet/vegans
animosity directed towards
243–6
athletes 166
city dwellers and 97–8
'extremists', labelled 1, 15, 241
food alternatives 217–20
media and *see* media
'propaganda' 2–3, 229, 262
talking about 233–51
term coined 262
Veganuary 209, 224
vegetarianism 9–10, 16, 20, 67, 73,
151, 160, 178, 193, 207
Venus flytrap 22
vertical farms 259
vitamins 165
B6 174, 175
B12 161, 172–3
C 167

D 41, 170, 174, 175
K 169

Waal, Frans de 19
water pollution 98, 119–22, 126,
127
Watson, Donald 262
Watters, Jesse 225–6
Waugh, Alison 208–9
Weber, Gary 151
wet markets 142, 143–4
Whacon 201
whaling 124–5, 155, 162,
201, 240
white veal 68–9
Whole Foods 222
wholefoods 163–4, 174, 176, 177,
178, 185, 186
wild animal trade 131–2, 133,
146, 148
wildflower meadows 256
Williams, Venus 166
woodlands 101, 256, 257
World Health Organization
(WHO) 129–30, 144, 154,
155, 156, 182, 211
World Organisation for Animal
Health (OIE) 130
Wye, River 121–2

yellow fever 146
Yorkshire 97, 99

zero-grazing systems 66